Kefir Milk

How to Ferment and Make Your Own Kefir Milk the Healthy Way

(Enjoy This Probiotic Drink with Dairy Free and Alternative Kefir Recipes)

Michael Burke

Published By **Phil Dawson**

Michael Burke

Kefir Milk: How to Ferment and Make Your Own Kefir Milk the Healthy Way (Enjoy This Probiotic Drink with Dairy Free and Alternative Kefir Recipes)

ISBN   978-1-998901-70-8

Legal & Disclaimer

The information contained in this book is not designed to replace or take the place of any form of medicine or professional medical advice. The information in this book has been provided for educational & entertainment purposes only.

The information contained in this book has been compiled from sources deemed reliable, and it is accurate to the best of the Author's knowledge; however, the Author cannot guarantee its accuracy and validity and cannot be held liable for any errors or omissions. Changes are periodically made to this book. You must consult your doctor or get professional medical advice before using any of the suggested remedies, techniques, or information in this book.

Table of Contents

Chapter 1: Your Gut: Take Care Of It and It Will Take Care Of You.

Do you suffer from digestive issues like diarrhea constipation, abdominal pain gas, bloating, stomach pain? Are you suffering from fatigue and fatigue? Do you tend to be a victim of everything happening? Do you suffer from yeast infections? Are you suffering from allergies? or have your current allergies become worse?

As soon as you're born, bacteria begin to colonize your gut via exposure to the microflora of your mother and the surroundings surrounding you. This is good! The bacteria have an intimate relationship with your body. It takes care of them and they care for you.

Your digestive system is home to between 300-1000 species of beneficial bacteria, named "gut" or "microintestinal" flora.

They help to maintain the health of your intestinal linings. They help with digestion, block the development of harmful bacteria, create important vitamins and hormones that help fight allergies and aid in regulating your immune system.

But, many factors can disrupt healthy bacteria within your system, such as serious illness, yeast or other parasites broad-spectrum antibiotics toxic environmental pollutants and even your diet, for example, consuming excessive amounts of alcohol, sugars, and carbohydrates. The gut flora could affect the effects of antibiotics administered to the animals that served as the last dinner.

If beneficial bacteria colonies die or are destroyed, yeast and bacteria that are harmful are able to thrive. This could cause or worsen digestive issues like diarrhea and irritable bowel syndrome ulcers, inflammatory bowel diseases as well as chronic inflammation of the stomach. It may also cause periodontal disease and tooth decay and acne, vaginal infection, and allergies. In addition, when your body struggles to fight an overflow of harmful bacteria, it drains the energy you require to carry on your daily routine.

How do you replace beneficial bacteria and improve the balance of microflora within your digestive tract to attain optimal well-being and health, gain your energy back, and begin feeling healthier? The answer is found within "probiotics," which contain beneficial live bacteria, the most well-known among them is the Lactobacillus Acidophilus. Probiotic supplements are available to help you get on the road to better health, or improve the gut flora by adding probiotics-rich and nutritious foods to your daily diet.

Chapter 2: Probiotic Foods Have a Rich History

Most cultures have created probiotic-rich food items as a method to prolong the shelf life of food items. Sauerkraut, yogurt, miso, kimchi and natto buttermilk, pickled vegetables and kombucha, as well as kefir. All of these probiotic-rich food items are created through fermentation processes that depend on microorganisms to extend the lifespan of food items, alter their taste, get rid of harmful nutrients, and cut down on cooking time (and thus the amount of energy required to cook). These foods are great for improving gut health and will provide the most benefit by eating a variety from a wide variety frequently.

However, when you buy the majority of these items from the grocery stores of today typically, you won't get the health benefits from probiotics you have hoped for. The government's regulations and the need to extend shelf life (and profits) means that a lot of these items are pasteurized (or sometimes "ultra pasteurized"). High-temperature quick-time (HTST) pasteurization eliminates 99.9999 percent of microorganisms that are viable both bad and good.

So, when you're looking for foods that contain probiotics It is essential to read the labels carefully and ensure that the term "pasteurized" doesn't appear. Be aware that if you pick things from the canned goods department--anything that is bottled or jarred to be stored without refrigeration--it is likely to be pasteurized as a part of the process of canning. When you're located in the refrigerated area there's a chance you'll be more fortunate (there is one brand of sauerkraut I've found within an hour's driving distance of my house that isn't pasteurized) But don't rely on it.

The most effective way to increase the effectiveness of probiotics in foods and ensure that you're getting the finest ingredients is to create your own. The good news is that fermented or cultured food items aren't difficult to make! All you need is the right--inexpensive--ingredients, a glass container and a little patience to allow nature to work its magic.

Chapter 3: Have a Drink on Me: Fermented Probiotic Beverages

Fermented beverages are among the most simple methods to begin making your own effective probiotic and probiotic-rich foods. When people think of beverages that are fermented they envision wine and beer. Although both have been found to have health benefits when taken moderately, neither is especially potent probiotics. To maximize the effectiveness of probiotics You might want to think about some of the "k" beverages: kombucha or fermented tea or Kefir (pronounced "keh-FUR" or "keh-FEER," or, more often "KEY-fur," like Donald Sutherland's most well-known son) It is a highly adaptable cultured milk or juice.

Kefir was first discovered more than thousand years ago among the Ossetians from the Caucasus Mountains, where shepherds discovered that the milk they stored in their leather pouches could sometimes ferment into the form of a bubbly drink. This may sound like commonplace beginnings however there is a mystery surrounding Kefir.

The beverage is made up of what's called "kefir grains," which aren't actually grains in any way. When used (though they are able to be dried to store) Kefir grains look like little cauliflower florets. They're tiny colonies composed of over 35 different varieties of probiotic bacteria, yeasts proteins, lipids, and sugars. It is impossible to make milk kefir grains from scratch. As to how they became a reality at all in the first place...no one knows.

The 'Grains of the Prophet' were believed to have been given by the Orthodox people from The Northern Caucasus by Mohammed, as well as the necessary knowledge to make the kefir. As it was believed the potency of kefir could decrease if it was made popular, kefir grain was considered to be part of the family's wealth, passed down from generation to generation, and were kept for centuries as a secret that was kept under strict guard.

In the 1800s, Russian doctors discovered the beverage and its health benefits and began to use it to treat tuberculosis, as well as stomach and intestinal illnesses. First scientific research studies of the benefits of kefir for health were published towards the close of the century. However, they did not do any to benefit the general population Kefir grains were highly guarded and hard to obtain, so producing commercially kefir became a challenge.

If the story of the origins of the kefir grains is still a mystery, the tale of how it came to mass production is an epic fairy tale including the minor Russian prince, kidnapped fair maiden as well as an adventurous rescue.

Chapter 4: The Prince's Almost-Wife

It began with it being the All Russian Physician's Society. With the intention of making kefir accessible to their patients the members of the society reached out to two brothers, who had been businessmen. They had among other businesses an Moscow dairy. The Brothers, Nicolay Ivanovitch Blandov as well as Vladimir Ivanovitch Blandov, also owned holdings within the Caucasus Mountains, including a cheese production facility located in Kislovodsk.

If the brothers could get these grains, they wouldn't be able to only make Kefir at an industrial scale. They would as the only commercial producers, be able to have an exclusive access to the market for kefir.

According to the legend, Nicolay sent one of his employees, the beautiful and gorgeous Irina Sakharova to beg Prince Bek-Mirza Barchorov the local prince of the region of Kislovodsk in order to persuade the prince into offering her some grain. ("Kislovodsk," by the way, translates to "sour waters"--if you've ever had the pleasure of trying Kefir, a delightfully tart and tangy beverage, you might wonder whether it has anything to be to the title.)

Since kefir grains were thought of as to be a sacred gift from Mohammed, the prince Barchorov did not want to be a target for his people for breaking an obligation of the religion by handing any of them to someone else.

Convinced that their reason was lost, Irina and her escorts began their journey back home.

But the prince, unable to let go of the kefir grains, was unable to let go of his gorgeous new friend. He ordered his men to kidnap her, a bizarrely accepted practice in the realm of the prince at the time - with the aim of compel her into marriage.

When they learned of the situation of Irina after hearing about her plight, the Blandov brothers employed agents to orchestrate an enthralling rescue of the princess who was to be. With the assistance by the All Russian Doctor's Association, Irina along with the Blandovs were able to have Prince Barachov taken before the Tsar Nicholas II. The love-sick prince was dismissed from the case and was then ordered to pay compensation. He offered jewels and gold however, all Irina along with the Blandovs really wanted -- and what judge eventually decided to require Prince Barchorov to pay - was the smallest amount of grain of kefir.

Kefir was then available to the public for sale within Moscow around 1908. The majority of the kefir grain that are available out of the Caucasus region of today come from Irina's grains. However, another type with smaller grain sizes, that originated in Tibet is also located.

Kefir that is produced commercially, even though it's a tasty but not always authentic drink, leaves a lot to be to be. First , it's processed, and if low fat dairy or flavorings are utilized, it may contain a lot of sugars during the fermentation process. Additionally, it could contain unwanted additives. In addition, commercial kefirs are made using starters instead of the kefir grains. This means that commercial kefirs share more common with buttermilk than traditional kefir.

(You might be thinking about yogurt's health benefits of live bacteria is frequently proclaimed in commercials But isn't all commercially produced yogurt pasteurized? Yes! Since pasteurization kills living bacteria producers include more later. This is the same for vitamin C that is produced in commercially-produced orange juice. This is why fresh juice is always the best: even though there is some benefit by "added nutrition," micronutrients that are derived from the original foodsource, unaltered is the most potent source for your body as well as your overall health.)

Chapter 5: Kefir Cautions

Due to the abundance of beneficial bacteria present in the kefir, it's recommended to start drinking just a few inches of water per day. Doing too much kefir before your digestive system has had the chance get used to different levels of bacteria may result in similar digestive issues, like cramping and abdominal pain that you were trying to help ease. Once your body is adjusted and you are ready to indulge in kefir and enjoy it! It's delicious and is quite satisfying.

If you begin your journey with Kefir, you might also be suffering from flu-like symptoms for a couple of days while your body undergoes what's called an "healing crisis," a result of the process of detoxification.

Keep in mind that probiotics are living microorganisms that can cause difficult to treat diseases, such as lactobacillus septicaemiain those with compromised or weak immune systems, which includes infants and children as well as the elderly and people who are seriously ill. Talk to your doctor about the possibility of using probiotics for any of these categories, and in the case of pregnancy or nursing.

However, it is important to remember that people have been eating fermented and cultured foods since the time humans have been around. (Natural fermentation has existed long before homo sapiens. For instance, fruit can be fermented on its own when it is removed out of the branches, for example.) Probiotics aren't harmful for healthy individuals and moderate consumption shouldn't be a problem for older people and children It's only in dosages that are therapeutic (or excessive amounts (let's face it: homemade yogurt or kefir is delicious!) which is why caution is recommended.

Furthermore, properly fermented Kefir that has an acidity of less than 4.5 and can prevent or stop the growth of many microorganisms that cause illness. But it does not stop the growth of Escherichia-coli, Listeria monocytogenes, Salmonella spp. or Yersinia enterocolitica. It is essential to start with kefir made of high-quality ingredients to prevent contamination with these pathogens in the first place.

If you're looking to be sure that your kefir is "properly fermented," you can buy pH test strips for sale at a reasonable price at health food stores, pharmacies shops and gardens stores (where they're used to test soil). Be sure to purchase strips that are lower than 4.5 pH.

Chapter 6: Making Kefir: Dairy, Coconut, Other Milks & Water

Dairy Kefir

The most popular type of kefir is comparable to yogurt and buttermilk. It is also sour cream and other milk-based products. However, there is also a tasty "water" kefir that can be made with sugar juice, water and coconut water. These are the types of kefir we'll discuss in this article. The dairy-based kefir grains include a diverse flora comprised of lactic acid bacteria that include lactobacilli and lactococci, as well as leuconosto. These bacteria are not just able in recolonizing your gut flora but also cause overgrowth, and eradicate or overwhelm the populations of harmful bacteria including ulcer-causing H. the pylori bacteria (which is also associated with the risk for stomach cancer).

Additionally, kefir grains are the only ones that can "unlock" peptides that are tied (or "encrypted") in milk. These peptides may help reduce blood pressure and boost cholesterol levels, boost your immune system and encourage more efficient digestive digestion for proteins.

Kefir is also high in biotin as well as vitamins (B12 B1, B1, and Vitamin K) as well as minerals (calcium magnesium, potassium and the phosphorus) along with the amino acids essential to life (proteins) like tryptophan.

Similar to buttermilk and yogurt Kefir is rich and creamy, and also is a refreshing tangy taste to it. Differently from buttermilk and yogurt, kefir is carbonated at the very least.

Despite being made of milk, kefir, which is a source of lactase, an enzyme which reduces lactose, can be absorbed by lactose intolerant people. In fact it has been shown to help reduce symptoms of maldigestion due to lactose including gas, bloating, and stomach pain up to 70 percent. You can also make use of rice, soy, or nut milks to make your own kefir.

In closing dairy kefir grains may be combined together with coconut milk to create an extremely thick, rich and extremely healthy cultured cream.

There are many other useful and free software available in the Download page that you may also take advantage of. Additionally, there is additional information that may be of use.

"Water" Kefir, or Tibicos

Kefir made from water, referred to as tibicos, tibi Japanese crystals of water, California honey bees and sugar kefir, can be all over all over the world, with every culture having its own unique spin on it.

Like other grains of kefir they are a form of bacteria, primarily Streptococcus and Lactobacillus Pediococcus and Leuconostoc as well as yeasts.

Water kefir can be a wonderful alternative for people who want to stay away from dairy products. It's also refreshing and a fantastic economical and healthy alternative to soft drinks.

Making Dairy-Based Kefir at Home

The first step to make the kefir at home is getting the grains for kefir. Be sure to purchase grains, not starter. If you take care of your grains with care then you won't need to buy grains again In fact the grains will grow and you'll have the ability to take the excess to families and friends, similar to like starters made from sourdough. The most efficient method of finding Kefir grains is to conduct the Internet search. You can try "live kefir grains" in Google. You'll see milk and water kefir grains.

There is no need for a huge amount of grains in order to start--as as little as a tablespoon will make a serving, and the kefir grains will increase with time which will allow you to create bigger batches. There's no need for expensive equipment. A glass jar, stainless steel, plastic bamboo, or cane strainer and wooden or plastic spoon or spatula made of rubber will suffice for your job. Simply add milk and you're ready to go! It's very simple.

Milk Kefir Recipe

Ingredients

2 cups of milk preferred organic, but is not a requirement for milk from cows (goat milk is a great alternative)

* 1-2 Tbsp milk kefir grains

Instructions

1. Make sure to fill a clean, pint-sized glass jar with milkand leave at least one-half inch headroom.

2. Include the Kefir grains.

3. The jar's opening should be covered by using a clean, dry cloth or coffee filter that is secured by the elastic of.

4. Place the jar on your counter or put it in a cabinet for 12 to 36 hours. It will thicken and form clumps as the majority of the grains of kefir can be seen rising to the surface. (If you let it sit for long enough, it'll separate in the clear fluid (kefir-whey) and then clumps (curds)--don't throw it away; it's still a great batch!) After about eight hours of fermentation, lightly shake the jar occasionally to help the fermentation process in absorbing all of the milk. The longer you continue to ferment your kefir, and the more grains

you add, the more sour it gets. You'll need to experiment to determine the amount of culturing that's the most pleasing for your taste.

5. If it's thickened enough and has becomes clumpy, stir the mixture with an wooden spoon or spatula. Pour it into a strainer set in a glass bowl Jar. Stir the kefir through the strainer to ensure that it goes through leaving only the grains.

6. Pour fresh milk into an unclean glass jar and add the grains. sprinkle a bit of the kefir that you have just removed then your next batch is in the making!

Then you'll be presented with the Jar (or bowl) of delicious Kefir. There are several options in your hands: You can drink the kefir right away. It can be put in an airtight container or bottle and store it in the fridge. It can be placed in an airtight container or bottle, and let it sit in the refrigerator for another couple of days for it to "ripen," then chill it in the fridge until you're ready to drink. While the kefir sits it becomes more nutritious (and tasty) and bio-synthesis produces vitamin B6, B3, and B9.

You may be wondering about the reason step 6 of the recipe is to add some of the fermented kefir into the batch you're about to start. This is known as "continuous fermentation." The Kefir's kefir vapor instantly reduces the pH of fresh milk, causing it to become acidic and stopping the growth of undesirable bacteria that could be present in the milk.

Tips

The more warm your kitchen is will be, the quicker the milk will start to grow. The longer you let it to rest and get more cultivated it will be. In addition, the more grain added, the quicker and more it will be able to develop.

For a more thick kefir you can substitute part of your milk with. The more cream you add, the thicker the result. It's possible to get the consistency of yogurt.

Coconut Milk Kefir

A good alternative to dairy the coconut milk is rich of medium chain fatty acids (MCFAs) along with monolaurin, which help boost your body's immune system. Kefir that is a result of this is extremely dense, and is better suited to smoothies and parfaits instead of drinking by itself.

It could take a batch or two to make your milk kefir grains are adapted to coconut milk. Moreover, it's suggested to soak the grains in regular milk every now and then to keep them healthy and content.

Ingredients

* 1 can of unsweetened, full-fat coconut milk

* 1 Tbsp milk kefir grains

Instructions

1. It is best to pour (and scoop) the coconut milk into a glass pint-sized jar. Mix to combine the watery part of the coconut milk the solids.

2. Add the grains to the bowl and gently stir until they are combined.

3. Clean a paper towel or coffee filter across the opening of the jar and secure it with the elastic band.

4. Place it either on the counter, or within the cupboard for 12 to 36 hours, examining often within the first 12 hours.

5. The removal of the grains is tricky with coconut milk compared to regular milk, due to the thicker consistency of Kefir that

results. You might have to look to locate the grains. If you do find the grains make use of them to begin another batch or follow the steps to store them.

The coconut kefir should be stored in a jar that has a lid. It should be stored within the fridge. It is not advisable to put it out on the counter since the kefir will ferment for a long time, which can make it too sweet.

Other Milks

Soy and nut milks perform well when added a bit of sugar to the fermentation. The grains need to be treated the same way as those with coconut milk. Soak in milk at least once a week to refresh them and boost healthy growth.

Ingredients

* 2 cups at room temperature soy, almonds rice, rice or another grain-based or nut milks

If you're using unsweetened "milk and cream,' you'll also require 1/8 cup of sugar (do not make use of sugar alcohols, honey, stevia, or sugar alcohols or artificial sweeteners)

* 1-2 Tbsp milk kefir grains

Instructions

1. Add the milk and, if you are using sugar, to an unclean glass pint container. Stir until the sugar has dissolving.

2. Incorporate the Kefir grains.

3. Place a coffee or cloth filter over the top of the jar. Secure by a band of elastic.

4. Allow to sit for 24 to 48 months on the counter in a cabinet. Make sure to gently shake the jar periodically within about 8

hours until the kefir has reached the level you want for fermentation.

5. Mix the kefir using a wooden spoon or a rubber spatula, and then pour the kefir through strainers into a fresh glass container.

6. Use the grains to store them or use them to start the next batch.

7. Enjoy your freshly brewed kefir or cover it and keep it in the fridge to use later.

Making Water Kefir at Home

The water kefir process requires a different type of grain unlike milk Kefir. These grains have a translucent appearance and change the color of the liquid , or the type of sugar you are using to ferment your Kefir. It is possible to use dairy kefir grains but because they're not receiving the nutrients the thrives on, they won't develop and, over time, stop producing entirely.

The grains of water kefir require nutrients to grow. Molasses, particularly rich blackstrap molasses can supply those minerals.

Numerous different sugars like cane beet, palm brown rice syrup, fruit, etc.--can be used to make your kefir with water However, you should steer clear of raw honey, as it contains bacteria that can cause adverse consequences for your grains. Also, beware of artificial sweeteners such as stevia and sugar alcohols (xylitol or erythritol.) since they're not fermentable. If you'd like to use the sweetener as a pure ingredient to your drink you can, however, when you are using them to replace sugar during the actual process of fermentation you won't get the kefir.

If you're concerned about the sugar that's added to your diet, remember worried: the sugar is meant to be used by the kefir, not for you. The final item will taste more acidic and sweet once fermenting has consumed most of the sugar. (If your kefir tastes sweet after fermentation with the grains, then you might have added excessive sugar, or not fermented for long enough, or perhaps your grains have been damaged.

Preparing the Water

Instead of being fermented in milk, the water Kefir grains are fermented in a mix of sugar and non-chlorinated waters. The non-chlorinated component is very crucial since chlorine kills the grains. If you have tap water that comes from a public source (as as opposed from well water) it is necessary to get rid of the chlorine first. This is fortunately, easy to accomplish and there are a variety of alternatives:

1. Fill a jar or bowl with water, then set them on your counters for up to 24 hours.

2. Bring the water to a boil that you'll use for 15 minutes.

3. Consider investing in a charcoal-based water filter, whether for your faucet or for a pitcher-based.

Basic Recipe for Water Kefir

This recipe requires you'll be fermenting pure sugarwater. It is best to gain a feel about this method before moving on to more complicated recipes that require adding the water kefir grain to the juices and other liquids. Kefir grains will develop easily, which will allow you to put some backup grains aside before moving into fermenting other liquids. That way, in the event that something goes wrong and your grains suffer it's not in danger of losing your kefir.

If you've been hoping to add the addition of fruit or other flavors to the first attempt at kefir Do not despair. With the recipe's basic formula you'll still be able to have plenty of flavor the second phase of fermentation when the grains are removed.

Ingredients

• 6 cups non-chlorinated non-chlorinated water

A 1/3 cup sugar

* 1 teaspoon blackstrap Molasses

* 1/3 cup of water Kafir grains

Instructions

1. Make a mixture of 1 cup of the water with the sugar together in a saucepan at medium-low heat. Stir until the sugar is completely dissolved.

2. Let it cool for about 10 minutes. Pour into a half gallon glass jar, and add five more cups of water as well as the Molasses. Mix to distribute the molasses.

3. Once the mixture is cool to ambient temperature, add the rice kefir water grains.

4. Use a clean, dry paper or coffee filter along the opening. Secure it by the help of a rubber band.

5. Keep it in a warm area for up to 24 hours or until you see bubbles (tiny carbon dioxide molecules) after you shake the container.

6. Place a mesh strainer (not aluminum) over a half-gallon glass jar . Pour the kefir mixture from one jar to the next, separating away the grains.

Chapter 7: Kefir Troubleshooting

While kefir is easy to make and doesn't require anything to worry about but there are a few points to look out for.

Flat and/or Sweet Kefir

Kefir is supposed to have at the very least some carbonation, with a tang of sour. If your kefir is dry and sweet (or it is, for dairy kefir, it tastes similar to milk rather than like yogurt) it could be due to a range of factors:

1. It wasn't fermenting for long enough. Kefir is more difficult to ferment in colder temperatures. What might require a couple of days on the counter in the summer heat could take three days during the middle of winter. If you've already taken out your grains from the jar, then you'll have to start from scratch. If you're tasting with the grains within the liquid

cover the jar, and let it remain for another couple of days.

2. Your grains aren't performing their job. If you've just recently stored grains in your pantry, they might remain dormant. Create a few more batches and observe how they develop over time. Don't consume any of the batches until you can produce an alcohol-like liquid that has an unmistakably sweet, fresh, and perhaps a slight yeasty smell. If there is no fermentation, there is always the possibility that your product may contain pathogens.

3. If you're making water kefir, you might start with too much sugar--the ferment process is only able to consume so much over a period of time. You may also have used sugar as a sweetener instead of sugar. Artificial sweeteners like stevia and sugar alcohols like erythritol and xylitol

won't nourish your grains and will not ferment into the kefir.

Water Kefir: Slime, Film, Bad Smells and Shrunken Grains

If your kefir grains are slimy, kefir is smelling like sulfur stinky feet, decaying fruit, or If your kefir appears to be thick or has an opaque white film over it or if the grains are shrinking instead expanding, your grains could be stressed, dehydrated or infected. Fortunately, you'll be in a position to bring them back to life with just a bit of the kefir grains "spa treatment."

In this case, you'll would like to keep your grains in a tummy So, you should purchase two four quarts of filtered or spring water. (If you happen to have spring water available on the tap, you could use this instead.)

Bring one quart of water to an end of boiling and then set aside.

In a glass jar that is quart-sized In a glass jar, mix the following:

* 4 tablespoons of granulated sugar (the less refined , the more refined)

* 1/2 tsp of unsulfured blackstrap Molasses

* 1/4 tsp baking soda

* 1/8 teaspoon sea salt

* 1 tablespoon cleaned oyster shell (available at any place where Aquariums are available)

Pour the boiling water in just a few inches from the top container. Stir until all the other ingredients are dissolving. Allow to cool to the temperature of room.

While you wait for your mixture to chill in the refrigerator, fill a small container with another one quart of water. The grains should be placed into a strainer made of plastic and then place the strainer into the water bowl so that the grains are able to be bathed in. Mix the grains with your fingers. It's okay to rub them against the strainer just a little as it helps to remove any debris that may be sticking to the grains' surface. Rinse the water off and then repeat the process with a fresh bowl of water. Repeat until you've used the whole second quarter of a quart.

Once the mineral solution, water, or sugar solution, has been cooled to room temp then you can add the grain. Cover the opening using a lid or the plastic piece stretched across the opening, and then secured with the elastic bands.

Then, place the jar into the refrigerator , allowing your grains time to sit for 3 or four days. (They can be kept in the refrigerator with this way for upto two months , if you do not have time to put them ready to go soon.)

If your grains have had enough rest, they will be healthy and fresh. If they're still slimy, or if the smell isn't gone you can repeat the treatment.

If you've got healthy-looking grains, make a new batch of molasses and sugarwater by using the standard water Kefir recipe. Separate the grains from the resting solution and begin your first batch of water kefir.

Milk Kefir: Slime

It's normal. It is produced through the polysaccharide soluble called kefiran which is a component of the process of milk kefir. Temperatures that are warmer and the different milk types could trigger an increase in the production of this chemical.

Milk Kefir: Foul Smells, Lack of Grain Growth

A milk kefir fermenting in a new way that is sour or has a bad smell, or grains that don't grow as fast (or in any way) could indicate the grains may be stressing. Relaxing can help them recover. Follow the steps for storing your grains in a story for up-to a week. This is found in the section storage and "resting" your kefir grains.

Mold

If you spot tiny floating circles around the outside of the kefir which appear like the mold you've seen on food items in your fridge Then you've got what you're thinking of is mold. There are several possible causes:

Contamination - If there is contamination present when you prepare your kefir for fermentation, or in the beginning stages of the kefir's fermentation with more acidity that can encourage the development of mold. Make sure to use clean, sanitized vessels and utensils. Clean hands, and high-quality ingredients for making the kefir.

Insufficient fermentation - If your Kefir was not fermented enough--or if the pH was not lower than 4.5--it won't be sufficiently acidic to stop mold growth.

To ensure your safety to avoid harm, it is recommended to get rid of any batch that has been affected by mold. Inspect the kefir grain; If they've become damp, you should get rid of them. If the grains do not appear to be affected, wash them thoroughly in chlorinated but non-chlorinated water. Check the subsequent batches for any signs of mold.

Fruit Flies

If you're fermenting your kefir using the lid, you should not experience this issue. It's also unlikely if you're using a cloth or a coffee filter that is secured to the mouth of the jar. Not likely but is possible. If you notice fruit flies in the jar, but they haven't made it into the jar, take the jar from its location and take off the coffee filter or cloth that covers the opening, then clean the exterior of the jar, and the inside of the opening thoroughly and secure a new material or coffee filter to the opening.

If you see any flies in the jar take the batch out clean your grains and begin with a new, clean container.

Chapter 8: Caring for Your Grains

Don't allow your grains to come into proximity to aluminum. Steel is fine however, to ensure the highest chances of ensuring the health of your grains, you must limit even that to the extent feasible: a stainless steel mesh strainer which your grains will only interact with for a couple of minutes at a stretch, won't have the same impact as the process of culturing your Kefir in stainless steel bowls.

Although it's essential to make sure you use a clean container each time you begin making a new batch, it's equally crucial to not put your grains in the jar that is hot. Make sure to cool your jar to room temperature after you've cleaned it. Injecting milk to the glass prior to adding the grains can help to ensure that the glass will not become too hot.

Storing or "Resting" Your Kefir Grains

There is a chance that you don't wish to commit your (entire) duration of your life to cranking out batches of kefir. Kefir grains are sturdy enough to allow you to take breaks of anything from a few hours or even 18 months. It is also possible to utilize these methods to keep surplus grains. These are the options available:

Taking a Break for up to a Week

Place your grains in an ice-filled glass jar and add the exact amount of milk you typically use to make Kefir. Cover it with a lid and then place it in the fridge. This method can keep your grains for upto a week.

Taking a Break for up to Two Months, Method #1

Follow the steps to take a break at least a week, and then follow them again with a new batch of milk each week. Do not exceed two months, or you risk getting your milk slowed down or even damaging the grains you've been eating.

Taking a Break for up to Two Months, Method #2

It is similar to similar to the "up to one week" method, however in this instance, instead of changing the milk each week, you begin with a larger amount of milk, and let it to run. Each week that you don't intend to use the grains, you should add at minimum 30 percent more milk into the container. For example, if, for instance, you normally produce two cups from milk then for each week that you plan to store your grains you'll add 0.6 cups (4.8 fluid ounces) of milk. If you want to store your grains for four weeks you'll need 3.8 cups (the two cups originally for a week and 0.6 multiplied by three weeks). Round the total to 4 cups, even and more milk will not hurt however less is not recommended.

Taking a Break for up to Two Months, Method #3

If you don't wish to replace the milk each week, and don't want to keep the milk in a large container in the refrigerator (if you usually make one quart of kefir it would require one gallon of milk in order to keep your grains for two months in the method #2) You can store your grains in the freezer for up to 2 months.

To do this, boil water in a pot for three minutes in order to make it sterile, and then let the water completely cool. (Very important!) It is essential to wash your grains in cool water and then gently dry them in white towels that have been sterilized. It is possible to sterilize the towels through ironing. Be sure they're fully cooled prior to using them to cover the grains.

Place the dry grains into the sealed jar or bag. If they're milk grains, sprinkle them with dry milk powder in sufficient quantities to cover the grains. The grains can be frozen for up to two months. (You can technically freeze grains for up to an entire year, but after two months, yeasts start to disappear and this will affect the general health of your grains.)

Taking a Break for up to 18 Months

For storage for the long term of kefir grains, wash the grains using the water which has been sterilized (by boiling for no less than 3 mins) and then cool completely. The grains can be dried by rubbing them between white towels that have been sterilized or let them air-dry while they lie in the towel. Also, you can clean these towels with irons, but make sure that they've been completely cooled before placing them to cover the grains.

To dry grains, you'll require a frame made of wood. An embroidery hoop is ideal for this job. Spread a clean piece nylon onto the hoop. A piece made from women's hosiery will work just fine. Put your grains onto the nylon, and then put a second layer on top of the grains to shield them from contaminates and insects. Place the hoop in a well-ventilated location and allow to dry until the grains are soft. This could take about a day or two for the water kefir grains that, once dry, may range from transparent to a light, crystal clear. For milk kefir grain, it could take between two and four days before they are completely dry. They tend to be yellowish.

When your grains are dry and stored within an airtight bag within the refrigerator.

Taking Your Kefir Grains out of Storage

Grain that is refrigerated

If you have grains that were kept refrigerated in milk once you're prepared to consume them just filter your liquid (which is actually Kefir, and food-safe) as per the standard procedure. Your initial batches may take longer than normal to ferment because the grains have been put into semi-dormant mode. When their metabolism gets up to speed and your culturing times resume normal.

Frozen grains

Restoring grains from their frozen state can take anywhere from two to three weeks. It could be longer. Begin by placing the grain in a glass that is filled with non-chlorinated water for about a couple of minutes to let them thaw. If they're milk grain which have been preserved in powdered milk that has dried and then rinse them in a strainer using non-chlorinated water.

After that you can add fresh milk to the milk-kefir grains or use your standard sugar-liquid recipe for water-kefir grains. However, instead of the typical ratio of liquid-to-grains ratio, you'll need to use just three times the amount of water as the grains. If you've got two tablespoons of grains, you'll only need six teaspoons liquid. Fill your container with water.

In the next 24 hours you can strain it out and then discard the liquid and replenish the liquid with new. Repeat this process until your milk grains reach complete coagulation (that forms clumps and whey) after 24 hours, or until your water grains have the ability to be carbonated. Whatever the case, the final product should have a clear and sour, perhaps slightly yeasty scent. This can take up to a week. Once you've reached this point, you should double the volume of liquid, and repeat the procedure until your grains reach complete coagulation in less than 24 hours. Then, increase the liquid in the same proportion until you are at your regular "production" quantity.

Dry grains

Rehydrate your dried grains using a container of suitable liquids Fresh dairy for milk kefir grain, or sugar water for grains of water kefir. Every day, you should remove the grains from the jar and then replace it with new until the grains can create a liquid that is cultured with an unmistakably sour, clean, perhaps yeasty smell in less than 24 hours. It can take between 4 to 10 days to attain.

Chapter 9: Kefir Recipes

Alongside a variety of water kefir-based recipes that are delicious This section also includes recipes for healthy cheese, yogurt salad dressings snack, smoothies, and desserts made with the kefir.

Drinks made from water that is already fermented Kefir

These recipes are based on water kefir fermented with simple sugar water. The sweetener is able to be used in these recipes as required however, you might enjoy them without. Because the process of fermentation is already completed it is not restricted to sugar-based sweetenerslike saccharin, xylitol and stevia etc. They can also be utilized.

Kefir Lemonade

* 1 one quart water kefir

1. 1/4 cup juice of a lemon

* Sweetener (optional)

* Mix the lemon juice. Taste, add sweetener if necessary.

Kream Soda

* 1 one quart water kefir

3 teaspoons of vanilla

Start with 2 teaspoons vanilla, mixed with 1 quart of Kefir. Adjust the vanilla according to required.

Cranberry Kefir

* 1 one quart water kefir

* 1/2 cup of cranberry juice

Mix water kefir with the juice of cranberries for an extremely delicious and healthy drink.

Kefir Soda

* 4 cups of water * 4 cups water for kefir

* 1 cup fruit juice

Combine the juice and kefir in the half-gallon container. (There is plenty of space left This is good because it prevents your container from burst when pressure builds up.) Put a piece or plastic wrap on top of the opening of the container, then screw or clamp the lid. Allow to sit at the room temperature for 2 up to three days before refrigerating. Enjoy cold!

It is possible to put the kefir mixture with juices into small bottles or even bottles and seal them. The process is similar let it the mixture sit on the counter at room temperatures for couple of days, chill, then drink.

Beverages that are made through the water kefir fermentation process

To make these drinks, mix the water kefir grains to any liquid other than sugar water, and let for them to ferment.

Coconut Water Kefir

* 1 cup coconut water

* 1 teaspoon Molasses

* 1/4 cup of water Kefir grains

Mix your coconut water with molasses into an oblong glass jar that is half-gallon in size. Add the Kefir grains. Wrap the kefir in a layer fabric or coffee filter, secured by an elastic strap. Leave at temperatures of room temperature for up to 24 hours. The kefir grains should be removed.

Zesty Citrus Kefir

Incorporate a few strips of organic lemon, orange grapefruit, lime or grapefruit zest into the base water Kefir recipe. The zest should be separated from the grains.

Juice Kefir

* 1 quart 100% fruit juice--try cherry, blueberry, grape, apple, etc. (Fresh-juiced

is recommended, if there is access to an juicer)

* 1 TSP Molasses

* 1/4 cup of water Kafir grains

Mix the molasses and juice in glass jars that are half-gallon in size. Add the grain of kefir. Then cover with a bit paper or coffee filter, and secure by an elastic strap. Leave in the room for up to 24 hours. The kefir grains should be removed.

Fizzy Ginger Lemonade

• 6 cups non-chlorinated, non-chlorinated drinking water

1 cup sugar

* 1 teaspoon Molasses

* 1/2 lemon

* One thin piece of of ginger and removed

* 1/3 cup of water Kafir grains

1. Mix sugar, water and molasses into a half-gallon glass jar. Attach the lid, to shake until the sugar is dissolved.

2. Add the ginger, lemon and kefir grains to mix well.

3. The lid is then screwed back. Set it on a table or in the cabinet for 24 to 72 hours, or until it has reached the degree of fermentation you're hoping for.

4. Get rid of the lemon and ginger out of the Kefir by pouring it through a strainer and into a large or smaller containers.

5. Close container container(s) and then let it rest at room temp for an additional 24 to 48 hours. Refrigerate for a few hours and then serve on the ice.

Kefir Yogurt

In the event that you replace some of the milk for cream while making your kefir, it is possible to create a thick, creamy Kefir.

Include sliced or pureed fruits coconut flakes without sugar and a squeeze of fresh lemon juice, and a sweetener to your yogurt made from kefir and you'll get an extremely healthy and nutritious snack.

You can also make Tzatziki (cucumber yogurt dip) Serve it with Mexican foods instead of sour-cream, or add some to your favorite soups or make it an ingredient in smoothies.

Kefir Cheese

Kefir is a great source of an incredibly soft, healthy cream cheese-like cheese. It's a must to have kefir that's fermented until the curds and the whey have been separated and the curds have grown quite thick, based on temperatures, grains and other factors the process can take up to up to 48 hours or more to attain this state.

After this recipe, there are a variety of recipes you can make your newly-created kefir cheese the kitchen, none of which requires cooking, which means you can keep the probiotic healthful microorganisms.

Four cups well fermented Kefir (Makes approximately. one cup cheese)

1. Cover a colander in plastic with a second layer of cheesecloth. Place the colander on top of an jar or bowl to collect the liquid whey.

2. Pour the kefir through the cheesecloth. Allow the kefir to go through the drainer in the fridge for between 24 and 48 hours.

3. Take the colander, kefir and bowl/jar from the fridge. Gather the edges of the cheesecloth, and twist the ends to form an sack, which has the curds from kefir in the bottom. Use the squeezer to pull more whey from the curds.

4. Let the cheese drain into the bowl. Scrape any cheese left onto the cheese cloth in the dish. Then you can add fruits, herbs and nuts, honey, nuts or even chocolate. Make your cheese in a log or ball and chill.

Note: You can use the whey for smoothies , or make use of it as an ingredient to ferment other food items: sauerkraut beets, homemade mayonnaise , Ketchup, etc.

Creamy Kefir Cheese Salad Dressing

* 2 Tbsp Kefir cheese

* 4 tablespoons fresh lemon juice

* 1 Tbsp milk

* 2 Tbsp fresh parsley, minced

* A pinch of cayenne

* Black pepper and salt

1. In a measuring cup that is liquid mix the cheese using the fork's back.

2. Add lemon juice slowly and stir to blend.

3. Mix in milk, parsley and whisk. Add the cayenne pepper and salt to taste.

Tangy Kefir Cheese Salad Dressing

* 1/2 cup of kefir cheese at room temperature

1 tsp of white wine vinegar

* 1 tsp Dijon mustard

* A pinch of powdered sugar

* 2 tablespoons of milk Kefir

* 2 Tbsp - 3 Tbsp water

* Black pepper and salt

1. 1 Tbsp chopped of scallion

1. In a measuring cup for liquids Mix together the vinegar, kefir cheese, powdered sugar and mustard.

2. Add the water and kefir, whisking until smooth. Add more water if needed.

3. Add salt and pepper according to your preference.

4. Before serving the dish, mix into the scallion just before serving.

Kefir Cheese on Apple Chips

Simple, quick and delicious dessert.

* One apple cut into slices

* A splash of lemon juice

* Kefir cheese

In a bowl, mix the apple slices with lemon juice to stop the slices from turning brown. Apply a small amount of Kefir cheese onto each apple slice, and then have fun!

Chocolate Kefir Cheese Truffles

The dates that are sweetened in the truffles contain dates, and are naturaland tasty treat that is simple to make as well! You can alter the sweetness of the truffle by changing the quantity of dates you choose to use.

* 10 Medjool dates, pitted

* 6 Tbsp of kefir cheese

1 cup plus 2 tablespoons sugar-free cocoa powder (try using a Dutch refined cocoa powder to make the most dark and rich of treats)

* 1 Tbsp vanilla

* A dash of salt

1. Process the dates using food processor.

2. Add cheese and 1/4 cup of chocolate powder, and salt. Process until the it is smooth and comes together in an elongated ball (approximately 20 minutes).

3. The rest of the cocoa powder can be placed on a platter or the small container.

4. Soak your hands in water and then cut off small chunks of the mixture of cheese and dates and make balls of them between your palms. Then, roll them in cocoa powder until it is dusty.

5. Keep it in the refrigerator for at least 30 minutes.

If you prefer to wrap the truffles in coconut flakes or chopped nuts, or try a few of both!

Kefir Smoothies

Between the milk kefirs Kefir yogurt, and water kefirs there is a huge palette to make delicious smoothies. Here are a few recipes to help you get started.

Very Berry

1. Cup milk Kefir (dairy or other)

1 cup frozen berries - you can choose to use all one variety or opt for an all-berry dessert

* 1/2 cup of ice cubes

* Add sweetener of your choice to taste

Mix everything except the sweetener in your blender . Let blend until the ice has been broken down and you've got yourself an ice-cream-like drink. Add sweetener as needed.

Pina Coolicious

1. 1 cup pineapple, cut into pieces

1. 1/2 Cup coconut milk Kefir

* 1/2 cup coconut milk

* 1/2 cup ice

* Add sweetener of your choice to taste

Mix everything except the sweetener in the blender. Blend until the drink is smooth. Add sweetener and taste as required.

Tropical Delight

* 1/2 ripe mango peeled, seeded and then cut into pieces

1 1/2 papaya ripe peeled, seeded and then cut into pieces

* 1 banana that is ripe, frozen (peel it prior to freezing)

• 3/4 cup water kefir either plain or fruit-flavored

* 1/4 cup regular or Kefir yogurt

* 1 teaspoon sweetener

* 1 cup ice

Mix all the ingredients in a blender, and blend until the mixture is smooth.

Pick-Me-Up Smoothie

* 1/2 cup of strong, chilled coffee

• 1/4 cup of milk Kefir (dairy or any other)

*1 1/2 cups of ice

* Sweetener can be added as an option to suit your taste.

All the ingredients, minus the sweetener to blend till smooth. Taste and adjust the sweetness.

Green Smoothie

* 1 cup of green grapes and frozen

1. A large apple not peeled, chopped into pieces

* 3 ripe kiwis, peeled

* 1 cup honeydew melon chunks

1-cup plain water Kefir, or coconut water Kefir

* A few spinach or kale leaves

* 1/2 cup ice

Combine all ingredients in a blender and blend until it is smooth.

Kefir Ice Cream

What a great treat for an incredibly hot day! You'll require an ice cream maker as well as some patience, because the mix must spend the duration of all day in the refrigerator before it can be transferred into the ice cream maker.

* 3 large eggs

*3 cups of cream

* 1 cup of milk Kefir

Two 1/4 cups milk

* 1/4 cup sugar

* 1 Tbsp vanilla

It's also necessary to have an aluminum half-gallon container that has lid.

1. Break the eggs into small bowls and gently beat them.

2. Add the eggs, cream, milk, and kefir into the container made of plastic. Mix until it is all combined.

3. Add vanilla, sugar, and sugar. whisk.

4. Cover the container with a lid and allow to sit within the fridge for up to 24 hours, mixing frequently to allow the sugar to dissolve.

5. Transfer the liquid into your Ice cream maker and follow the instructions to make Ice cream.

This recipe can be used to make a simple vanilla Ice cream. For different flavors, add extracts, fresh , or frozen fruits and chocolate shavings, nuts, syrup or other flavorings before you transfer the mixture to the Ice cream maker.

Kefir Popsicles

If you don't own an Ice cream maker Kefir popsicles are perfect for an incredibly hot day (or any time).

* 1 cup of kefir (milk or water)

* 1 lb. of fruit cleaned up and put through the food processor

* 1/4 cup honey

* 1 Tbsp vanilla extract

1. Mix the kefir, the fruit honey, vanilla, and kefir.

2. Try it out on your own. You'll want the flavor to be more sweet than you prefer since the freezing process will take away some of that sweetness.

3. Pour into popsicle molds.

4. Freeze.

5. Enjoy!

There are a myriad of possibilities to make variations with this one, in between the various types of kefir as well as the various fruits that are available: berries grapes, peaches, plums and pineapples. Your imagination is the only limit!

Kefir Fudgesicles

Fruit is nutritious, delicious and delicious and...sometimes it is just necessary to have chocolate. The tartness of cultured milk, such as cream cheese Greek yogurt and kefir, when paired with the chocolate's richness is a delicious and addictive combination. Try these and see if they don't meet your needs.

* 1 cup of milk or coconut milk Kefir

* 3 tablespoons of chocolate powder that is unsweetened (use Dutch processed for a dark, rich and dark treat)

* 3 Tbsp honey

* 1/2 tsp vanilla extract

* Sprinkle of salt

1. Mix all the components together.

2. Try it out on your own. You'll want the flavor to be a bit more sweet than you prefer since the freezing process will take away some of the sweetness.

3. Pour into popsicle molds.

4. Freeze.

5. Enjoy!

In place of vanilla make use of orange extract or peppermint. To make Mexican chocolate popsicles try the addition of a few drops of cayenne and cinnamon. Add toasted hazelnuts, or coconut flakes that have been toasted.

Chapter 10: Benefits Of Water Kefir

1.Rich in Beneficial Bacteria

A major benefit of drinking water kefir is the nature of its richness in probiotics. Probiotics are beneficial microscopic organisms found in the gut . it plays a vital role throughout the spectrum of wellness. It aids in stopping malignant growth , and also aids in to fight off. The evidence suggests yogurt as the main source of probiotics. Despite the fact that the sophisticated kefir is actually regarded as a premium source of probiotics. This is due to the fact that it offers a different variety of yeasts and microbes. In fact, some research indicates that kefir grains have over 50 distinct yeast strains and bacteria strains. These are the most frequent groups of gainful microbes that are found in kefir and they are

*Lactobacillus

*Lactococcus

*Streptococcus

*Leuconostoc

*Bifidobacterium

*Thermophilus

*Bulgaricus

*Helveticus

2.May Help Fight Cancer Cells

The test is confined to tests-tube considerations. This test recommends that water kefir may help in the prevention of certain types of malignancy. One of the test results that kefir's removal of toxins can be effective in preventing the growth of malignant cells in bosom. In the meantime, various tests conducted proved that kefir can be beneficial in fighting blood cancer as well as colon. This is evident because it is very rich in probiotics. It also assists in increasing the immune system, which can aid in the fight against malignant growth. However, there may be a the need to conduct further studies to evaluate this evidence.

3.Could Boost Immune Function

Due to the high concentration of beneficial microbes, the addition of water kefir to your diet every day will help boost your healthy, robust framework. Research and studies conducted on individuals showed that certain strains of probiotics may aid in reducing your risk of developing respiratory illnesses in addition to intestinal toxins and the likelihood of urinary tract infections among women. Research and studies conducted in animals demonstrated that kefir may help in the suppression of trigger reactions that are triggered by a variety of issues, including asthma.

A smaller study of six weeks conducted with 18 participants showed that drinking kefir every day could reduce irritation as well as increase the number of healthy cells within the body.

4.Dairy-Free and Vegan

The most common method of making kefir is using goat or cow milk mixed with Kefir grains. This produces a thick and probiotic-rich drink. However it is because the process of making water kefir using sugar water, it's an excellent option for those who opt to avoid dairy products, possibly due to personal health issues, or dietary restrictions. It's an excellent probiotics and for boosting your gut health when you are on the dairy-free or vegetarian diet, so that you can reduce your intake of animal things.

5.May Cause Side Effects in Some People

Kefir water can be enjoyed by a small number of individuals without the risk of adverse effects. However, there are frequent reactions that are associated to it include stomach-related issues, such as the appearance of swelling, queasiness, and even stoppage. The reactions disappear when the use is continued. People with fragile invulnerable structure, such as AID patients should consult their physician prior to using water Kefir.

6.Easy to make and enjoy at home

Water kefir is an awe-inspiring drink that is very easy to make. It comes with a number of health benefits that are beneficial in your overall health. Even though the flavor might differ due to of various factors, the best part about it is that it tastes a little sweet and has some lingering flavor.

Chapter 11: History Of Water Kefir

WHAT ARE WATER KEFIR GRAINS?

Some people are aware of milk kefir grains, but they are not water Kefir grains. It is important to note that both are made using "grains". In any event they aren't real grains, such as wheat or Rye. They are a collection of microbes, yeast and yeast living in a co-operative connection that is held by the polysaccharide (dextran) which is produced by the Lactobacillus higarii. The clumps of microbes, yeast and polysaccharide look like precious stones also known as "grains" of jam. These microbes as well as yeast that are present in the grains make use of sugar to produce carbon dioxide as well as lactic acid, and alcohol (limited amount).

SEVERAL NAMES FOR WATER KEFIR GRAINS

The grains of water kefir are known by many names. Most commonly, they are called Japanese Tibicos, water-based precious stones or California honeybees. They're also known as Australia Bees, Water Diamonds African bees Ginger Bees, Ginger Beer Plant to mention but there are a few. Water kefir is known by many different names across different countries. They are known as piltz Germany and are referred to as Kefir di Frutta from Italy and are referred to as Graines Vivantes in Mexico. The yeasts and microscopic organisms within the water kefir grain are active. It is essential to be aware the variety of the specific strain that produces that bubbly, water-kefir drinks.

ORIGIN OF WATER KEFIR

The exact location where the water kefir grains came from isn't entirely certain. However some theories suggest that it originated from Mexico. There is some evidence that the tibicos tibicos cult is developed on the stacks on the Opuntia desert plant can be described as hard granules, which could be reconstitued in a sugar-water arrangement in the form of growing Tibicos. There is evidence of the late 1800s in Mexico that mentions water kefir grains being used as a matured drink that was made with an improved juice from the pear that was thorny desert plants. There are a few accounts that put their origins or usage, in Tibet in and the Caucasus Mountains, the southern region in the Ukraine. The ability to pinpoint exactly in the history of water kefir is extremely challenging because water kefir societies can be found across the globe and no two communities are exactly the identical. There is no written historyof the water kefir, which is making it difficult to pinpoint a start time. Studies have revealed that these grains were extensively used over a long period.

Some names for water kefir.

* Tibicos (Tibi)

* Bulgaros

* Bees

* Japanese Water Crystals

* Japanese Beer seeds

* Graines Vivantes (French)

* Wasserkefir

* Sugar Kefir Grains

* Piltz, (German)

* Kefir di Frutta (Italian)

* Kefirs/Keefir/Kephir

* Aqua Gems

* Sea Rice

* Sugary Fungus

* Kefir d'acqua/water

* Kefir d'uva (grape juice is utilized)

* Bebees

* African bees

* California Bees

* Australian bees

* Vinegar bees

* Ginger bees

* Ale nuts

* Balm of Gilead

* Beer seeds

* Beer plant

Chapter 12: How To Use Water Kefir Grains

The method of utilizing water kefir grains is basically similar across the world , regardless of various names that are given to the grains of water kefir. They are generally used by adding sugar water to then allowing the process of life to develop for a few days to create a bubbly, aged drink.

SIMPLE STEP TO MAKE WATER KEFIR AT HOME

Combine 1/2 cup (118 milliliters) of water that is high temperature along by adding 1 teaspoon (50 grams) of sugar in a container or bowl.

Mix the mixture until it begins to break it down.

Add 3 cups (710 milliliters) of water at room temperature into the bowl or container.

Add your water kefir grain.

Cover and place the bowl the container or bowl in a sunny area that is heated to 68-

85degF (20 to 30 degrees Celsius) and allow to age for 24 for up to 48 hours.

*The next step is to separate those water-kefir grain out of the mix

*Add another batch of sugar water (the end product is prepared for you to use and enjoy).

*You may choose to drink the water kefir only for what it's worth or even add flavors, such as natural product juice vanilla concentrate, mint leaves or organic solidified products

Chapter 13: Medical Benefits Of Taking Water Kefir

1. Aids in the enactment of the Digestive System Water Kefir is a valuable ingredient in controlling the stomach's causticity , as well as in the action of the stomach related framework.

2. Helps to limit Food Intolerance

The water kefir is a good function to play in reducing food prejudice. Certain foods that believe they are difficult to digest don't circulate in the blood , rather they weaken digestion organs. This helps in assuming an immunological role, especially in the adjustment of microscopic organisms.

3. Aides Strengthens the Immune System

Water kefir can be a positive job to perform in a safe and secure environment. It is the lactic maturation that has antibacterial effects and could aid in providing our body with the protection it needs against illnesses and diseases. Probiotic microorganisms found in water kefir could help in controlling the over development of pathogens , as well as they break down microorganisms within the digestive system. Water kefir works as a natural disinfectant, and also aid in increasing digestion and the breath of cells.

4. Kefir-water is rich in Vitamins

Kefir water is a rich source of nutrients. It is rich with Vitamin C and nutrient B (B1 and B6). In addition, natural substances in water kefir also contain Vitamin C and other significant supplements.

The Vitamin B1

* Exercise cardiovascular capacity

*Improves cerebrum capacities

*Protects nerves.

*Assist in helping assimilation

*Protects the mucous layer.

*Prevents the development of pallor.

*Increases the amount of glucose.

The Vitamin B6

*It helps strengthen the resistance framework

*Helps improve mind capacity

*Helps improve our mental outlook

*Helps in treating hypertension.

* Helps prevent cardiovascular diseases.

*Helps to upgrade digestion

*Helps with the in the development of an enzymatic framework

Nutrient C

*Helps to reduce the incidence of asthma

*Helps prevent the occurrence of waterfalls.

*It helps to reduce levels of glycosylated hemoglobin

*Protects against the protein oxidation

*Helps in reducing the symptoms of chemotherapy for disease.

*Helps support a solid robust, secure framework

5. Diminishes Allergic Reactions

Probiotics present in water kefir could help with the prevention of sensitivities, as well as they fight microbes and diseases. The majority of sensitivities are caused by a fear of some kind of food consumed. The symptoms of hypersensitivity can alter from one person before moving to the next. Kefir water is extremely effective to reduce the risk of adverse reactions.

6. Water Kefir likewise assists with the development of energy levels

It is a good source of essential ingredients that boost the vitality of your body. By adding coconut juice to water kefir is a great way to assist to boost your energy levels, as coconut juice contains potassium that is beneficial in strengthening the muscles.

7. Water kefir is an anti-inflammatory user

The cause of irritation is injuries. The irritations are just a normal response of the body to hurt. In the event that there is a physical problem within the body or the body is injured it uses irritations to guard itself against the effects of microbes as well as infections. In order to do this effectively it requires additional supplements to aid in healing. When water kefir enters the body it is a good idea to take the minerals and microscopic organisms within the water kefir assist in providing nourishment to the body. Thus, water kefir is an excellent mitigating factor. Additionally, it helps heal certain ailments, such as like diarrhea, queasiness, and heartburn.

8. Battles Against Cancer

Drinking water kefir in moderation can aid greatly in fighting malignant growth. Studies and research have shown that drinking water kefir regularly can aid in the prevention of bosom and ovarian malignancies.

9. Water Kefir Act as an Anti-contagious and Antibiotic Agent

Drinking water kefir can be the best way to protect your body. Kefir water is a abundant source of probiotics which makes it an effective ally against parasites and anti-toxin experts. It also contains beneficial microorganisms that help it fight against a variety of illnesses and growths.

10. Forestalls Diabetes

Because water Kefir is a very bogat source of probiotics and probiotics, it is able to assist in reducing the level of sugar within the body. This makes it beneficial for those suffering from diabetes because it can help in stopping the blood glucose levels.

11. Treatment of Asthma

The water kefir refreshment can have an effective effect in treating asthma due to the proximity of reducing supplements.

12. Building Bone Density

Water kefir is a nutrient-rich source of manganese, calcium and magnesium that are vital in the process of reducing bone thickness. Research and studies have shown that drinking water kefir aids in enhancing bone thickness this way, decreasing the risk of developing osteoporosis. Kefir water can also aid in the storage of vital nutrients, such as calcium, phosphorus and nutrient D, and magnesium. Consuming water kefir regularly can help provide the essential nutrients needed for the development of strong bones.

Chapter 14: Types Of Kefir

There are two distinct varieties of Kefir. They are

1. MILK KEFIR

2. WATER KEFIR

*Milk Kefir: It's an anti-biotic beverage that is well-known and is available in many supermarkets.

*Water kefir is also a refreshing drink that is probiotic rich. It is crucial that it is not a source of dairy and has a light refreshment, and it can be improved the quality of your drink in various ways.

N.B. Kefir in both varieties possess distinctive qualities but they are produced in a surprising manner. If you're looking to include probiotics into your everyday routine and you are interested, take note of which of these beverages is most suitable for you.

DISTINCTION BETWEEN MILK KEFIR AND WATER KEFIR

Milk Kefir

Milk kefir is made from goat milk, bovine milk as well as coconut milk. It is also possible to make using other milks that are not dairy. It could result in the opposite result.

Water Kefir

Kefir water is created using the sugar-water mixture, natural juice, and kefir grains. Kefir water may also require the creation of a starter culture. It is possible to make use of an Kefir Beginner Culture or water Kefir Grains, it all depends on the frequency you'd like to make water Kefir.

WHAT KEFIR CONTAINS

Milk Kefir Grains are a customary starter culture which is used to make a probiotic rich drink that is made with live yeast and microscopic microorganisms.

Water Kefir Grains are also a common reusable starter culture used for dairy-free refined refreshment that is enriched with live active yeast and microorganisms.

HOW DOES KEFIR TASTE?

Milk Kefir

Milk kefir is a beverage with similar to that of refined milk. The taste of each kefir cluster, in all cases, is contingent on the rate of maturation. Kefir that has been aged for a long time may have a sharp, solid flavor and may be slightly carbonated. However, a slower aging time can provide a more delicate taste.

Water Kefir

Water kefir , on the other hand, is sweet, but slightly matured taste. Some people prefer improved water kefir.

STEP BY STEP INSTRUCTIONS TO FLAVOR KEFIR

MILK KEFIR

Milk Kefir is a great way to spice it by mixing it with the form of a solidified or new natural flavor concentrates or natural products like nectar, vanilla and Stevia, maple syrup and more. Some people prefer the process of maturing milk kefir over a further time to increase the quality and enhance.

WATER KEFIR

Water Kefir can then be spiced with new or dried organic products, concentrates to enhance like vanilla, herbs or even natural product juice.

DIFFERENT USES OF KEFIR

The Milk Kefir grains are used

*To vaccinate cream in order to create kefir cream or a refined spread.

The milk kefir grain could be used to create an initial culture for maturing vegetables.

* Extra milk kefir could also be used to cover flour prior to heating or baking sourdough.

Kefir Water Kefir is a great option to use in the following ways.

*It can be mixed with non-dairy milk to make non-dairy Kefir.

Extra water kefir grains could also be used as a an aging vegetable starter culture.

Extra water kefir may also be used as a boosting expert for the production of gluten-free starters for sourdough.

A Quick Look at the History of Water Kefir

The story of the origins of water Kefir, to my mind is fascinating. I'm not looking to go too deeply into the history of water kefir grains however, I believe it's essential to know the basics of the place they came from.

Where did the water kefir grains come from? The majority of information about the history of the water kefir grains is speculation.

Mexico appears to be the largest and most well-known area for these speculations. Beyond speculation, research conducted by M. L. Lutz in 1899 has documented the existence of the tibicos (water Kefir grains) within the Ountia Cactus. This cactusis often referred to as "the prickly pear", has a sugar-water environment where the tibicos thrives. Based on the study conducted by M. L. Lutz The tibicos develops over pad of cactus as hard, semi-translucent particles. The granules are harvested and then reconstituted by soaking them in an acidic solution of sugar and water. They then grow the sugar-water and result in water Kefir. The documents of the past mentioned the grains of water kefir were used in the production of a drink that was made by the juice that was sugary from the Ountia Cactus in Mexico.

Other sources and legends claim that tibicos might be a native of the Caucasus mountains or the southern part of the Ukraine as well as Tibet, China.

Here's a fascinating short story:

According to the legend, Mother Teresa of Calcutta went to the Himalayas and was given the water kefir grains of the Tibetan monks in order to distribute them among India's native people. The reason for this was to boost their health and alleviate them of ailments. The monks of the time had one rule: the grain of water kefir should not be offered for sale. They can only be distributed and shared at no cost! Mother Teresa also travelled to the Philippines with the water kefir grain for those Filipino people. What a cool idea!

We don't really know the exact origins of tibicos, and the chances are that we'll never find out. The task of determining the exact area or people that originated is more difficult because the grains of water kefir can be discovered all over the globe and no two cultures are exactly the same. Another obstacle in locating the origin of the grain is the absence of documented the history. When all the evidence is put together, it appears that brewing water kefir has been practiced for centuries. In addition to the place of origin of the practice, the method of culturing and fermenting the water Kefir is almost identical all over the world.

Health Benefits of Drinking Water Kefir

Water kefir is a drink that is a great source of health advantages. One of the most significant benefits of drinking water kefir could be the probiotic properties of the drink. We hear a lot about probiotics, but do you actually know what they are?

dictionary.com defines probiotics as: a product (such as a nutritional supplement) that contains active organisms (as lactobacilli) which is consumed orally to replenish beneficial bacteria in the body.

Probiotics are healthy and beneficial bacteria that help keep your gut healthy and happy. The gut is filled with over 1000 strains of beneficial bacteria. These beneficial strains of bacteria help to improve digestion improve the immune system and and keep our body healthy and in some instances could even help heal and help to prevent allergies!

There's been a myth that has been circulating for a while regarding water kefir being not more potent than other probiotic beverages, like Kombucha (fermented with black tea). This is a lie! Kefir water actually has an increased amount of probiotic strains that are more prevalent than kombucha or the other alternatives!

Injecting all these probiotic strains in your gut through the process of drinking water kefir can increase your immunity! If you have a stronger immune system it will reduce the likelihood of becoming sick.

Probiotics (water kefir and kombucha, as well as fermented foods) improve your immune system. It's true that 80percent of your immune system's strength is within the digestive tract.

Alongside these advantages in addition, the process of fermentation that occurs during the process of making water kefir produces a myriad of other vitamins and minerals. There aren't any chemical added, additives or any other substances in the water kefir.

The grains of water kefir will also last forever. That means that so long as you care for them they will take good care of you. Watch them expand and multiply.

My most loved benefit, aside from the probiotics and digestive health booster it's the ease of the entire procedure.

What You Will Need To Brew Water Kefir

It's quite obvious what is the primary ingredient is Tibicos!

It is essential to purchase top-quality water Kefir grains from a reliable source. As of now, I do not have any suggestions. In that regard please feel free to email my address at dab9416@gmail.com and I'll be able to offer one of two options to you: either send me some water kefir grain which I personally make using only premium fruit, sugars and water. If I don't have enough I'll go for a reputable source from which you can purchase top-quality water kefir grain from.

The second ingredient you'll require in order to make excellent water kefir that tastes delicious and high-quality is water!

In the present, I'm not sure the location you're currently in while reading this. I'm not sure which country you reside in or what your water sources are. I am within the United States. What I know is that you shouldn't to drink water that is of low quality. A good example of water that is not high-quality is that of the United States' water from the tap. There are a lot of undesirable elements that make up the tap water in the United States.

As an example the following substances are added regularly:

Fluorosilicic acid aluminium sulphateand calcium hydroxide and sodium silicofluoride.

Other chemicals that are commonly present in United States' tap water include:

Salts of mercury aluminum, lead Barium, radium copper, and cadmium. The fluorine compound, the nitrates chlorine trihalomethanes (THMs) pesticides, and hormones.

In this regard you've got a few alternatives: spring water coconut water well water, and the distilled water.

Personally, I suggest making use of high-quality spring water. Kefir water grains require minerals to flourish and reproduce. If you're using high-quality water from a spring, you don't need to be concerned concerning adding more minerals.

Kefir grains of water are usually thriving in well water because of its mineral content that is naturally high. Water from wells, depending upon the origin, could contain unwanted elements, like the high level of pesticides or iron.

Reverse-osmosis water is almost guaranteed to end up causing the demise of the water grain kefir. The reverse-osmosis water isn't enriched with enough minerals to enable the kefir water grains to flourish. You can try reverse-osmosis through the use of mineral. Be sure to keep an active grain of water kefir in good health and to have an emergency backup.

Water that is filtered can be used. A lot of people make their water kefir drinks with filtered water. I would advise you to inquire about what the purity of water filters you use and the water that is brewed. Water that is filtered can be deficient the mineral count. I will explore the issue of mineral content a bit more after we discuss the distilled water.

Utilizing distilled water can be an effective method. Distilled water has had the majority of its impurities eliminated through it being boiled before condensing it into a clear container. It is necessary to include minerals in distilled water to make water Kefir. In reference to the information we have discussed prior to this section the water kefir grains thrive in mineral-rich conditions.

Important: It's possible to increase the mineral content of the water you are using. I've not experienced this problem in my own drinking experience However, it's something you should be conscious of.

Here are a few ways that to mineralize water:

My absolute favorite is organic blackstrap molasses with no sulfur! Molasses is among the best ways to improve the mineral content of your water, and also encourage water kefir grains to expand and expand. Take note that the Molasses can impart a distinct taste to the water kefir drinks which you might or may not enjoy.

Certain people take mineral supplements (I have not tried this) with great success. Other options include sea salt that is unrefined, organic dried raisins natural citrus (or different citrus fruit) and eggshells that are of the highest quality.

Organically dried organic raisins as well as lemons from the garden are the few fruits that you can utilize in the brewing of water kefir in the beginning of the fermentation. There are also people who have enjoyed success with other fruits like limes and oranges. I suggest you wait until the second fermentation before you add your fruit. If you're planning include eggshells in your drink, ensure that they are from a reputable source. Local eggs that are fresh from the farm are the best option.

The various sugars you consume will aid in the mineral content of your water.

A third component in the water kefir recipe is sugar!

Sugar is an essential ingredient in the production of your water Kefir. Because the water kefir grains might differ, it could need some experimentation from your end. Your grains might react differently to different types of sugars that I suggest.

Here is my suggested list of sugars that you can test:

Pure cane juice crystals organic raw or turbinado sugar organic sucanat (or Rapadura) along with natural brown sugar (dark or light).

My personal favorite from my own experiences is sucanat and organic light brown sugar.

Remember that it's best to choose the finest sugars that are of the highest quality available. This implies that they are not processed at all and organic.

Here is my list of non-recommended sugars:

Sugar palm (coconut sugar) Honey, palm sugar (coconut sugar) or sugar substitute (stevia or splenda) as well as maple syrup or sugar and molasses on its own.

You can try small amounts of these sugars that are not recommended with the sugars that are recommended. Avoid using the sugar alternative honey. Honey is known to have strong anti-bacterial properties and could cause harm to the grains of water kefir. Sugar substitutes, however, aren't sugar. Kefir grains of water aren't able to be fed by sugar substitutes like the stevia. I recommend organic Stevia as a substitute for sugar in cooking, beverages and other uses.

There are other kinds of sugars that you might want to test. Here are a few examples:

Muscavado, Panela, Demarara powdered sugar, jaggery and sugar stalks of cane (swizzle sticks) piloncillo, and various kinds of sugars that are white.

I can't recommend these to anyone with a clear mind because I've had no knowledge of using these in my water Kefir. Don't be scared to try various sugars. Be sure to make sure you keep at the very least one pot of healthy water kefir grains that are alive and flourishing.

Yup, that's it! Three ingredients are needed to make water Kefir. Let's continue.

Brewing Your First Batch of Water Kefir

You made it! Let's go.

You'll need glass ceramic or food-grade plastic container of some type. I would recommend glass jars like mason Jars. They've always worked flawlessly for me.

Typically glass mason jars be a great containers for secondary as well as primary (if you decide to do that) the fermentation stages.

Beware: Avoid using any metal (besides stainless steel) in the brewing of water kefir.

Kefir water, as well as other substances that is acidic in nature, could cause leeching on metals. Steel made of stainless is fine. Making use of strainers made of stainless steel or stirring using the stainless steel spoon is not harmful to the water kefir you make. Make sure that the contact with stainless steel is only for a short time.

But, I would not recommend using the typical stainless steel lids for mason jars. If you do decide to use the lids, be sure to ensure that the kefir-water mixture get in contact with the lid during the fermentation process.

I suggest using plastic lids when feasible. In the initial fermentation process, it's okay to employ the cheesecloth or lid that is loosely fitted. The primary reason you cover the water kefir at the initial stage is to prevent contaminants from entering the container. It isn't necessary to seal the container sealed with air at this point.

Step One - Preparing Your Water Kefir Grains

If you got your water kefir grain from a relative who generously gave them to you, they're likely to be ready for use. If you bought them from an online store it could be dried grains or they could have been shipped by a sugar water.

Activating Dehydrated Grains

Warm up 3-4 cups of premium water to a high-quality temperature.

Dissolve around 14 cup of sugar in the water.

Incorporate your preferred form of mineral in the water.

Cool the sugar-water to a temperature that is around room temp.

Add the sugar and water to the container you have chosen.

Include all the dehydrated grains to the container.

Cover with cheesecloth and a rubber band or a loose fitting lid.

Set it in a warm place between 68deg and 85degF for 2-4 days.

After about 2-4 days after 2-4 days, your water kefir granules will be slender and transparent. You can dispose of the water used in the process of rehydrating and then give your kefir water grains the chance to rinse them with cold quality water.

Step Two - Culturing the Sugar-Water

It's time to make your first make a brew. Begin with a single brew, otherwise you could become overwhelmed and harm the grains of water kefir.

In order to cultivate a couple of quarters of sugar-water requires three or four tablespoons of water Kefir grains. I would suggest playing around with the ratios you use to determine the one that works for you.

The usual sugar ratio is 1/4 cup for each quarter quart. Again, I suggest using this ratio initially but don't be afraid of exploring.

Culturing Sugar-Water

Warm up a quarter cup of water that is high-quality and safe.

Dissolve approximately 14 cup of sugar in the water.

The sugar-water should be chilled until it is at or near room temperature.

Add the water to the container you have chosen.

Include 2-4 tablespoons water kefir to the container.

Incorporate your preferred form of mineral into the water.

Cover with cheese cloth and rubber band or loose-fitting lid.

Set it in a warm place that is between 68deg-85degF, for 24 to 48 hours.

If you let the water-kefir you have to grow the sugar-water for a longer period than this, they could become starved.

Be sure to watch your water kefir over the next 24 to 48 hours as it begins to ferment the sugar-water. It will start to show it bubbling and forming a ferment. You might notice that the kefir water grains are already starting to multiply or are floating up to the top. This is an amazing indicator!

It is an excellent option to brew. You can add sugar, however the water kefir grains should work just fine without sugar. It is recommended to culture the coconut water for 24 to 48 hours.

Step 3 - Straining Your Water Kefir Grains

Straining Your Water Kefir

Take the container filled with water kefir down to the sink.

Choose a mesh strainer of your you.

Then, gently pour the water kefir through the strainer and into an empty jar or container that is clean.

Put all your water kefir grains in an unclean jar or container.

There is now a container of water kefir that is finished. Continue Step 2 and then start the process once more. If the water kefir grains are already multiplying, you may begin two batches or one bigger batch.

It is possible to drink your water Kefir! The ideal drink is a mildly carbonated and tangy drink. Are you getting too sweet? Do you think it is too bitter? That's where the process of learning will begin.

You can decide to eat the kefir as it is or continue to flavor your water kefir with flavor, performing an additional fermentation, and creating delicious, fizzy drinks!

Secondary Fermentation - Making Delicious Fizzy Drinks

Here is where it gets exciting and fun. You've successfully learnt (and most likely created) the art of brewing water Kefir. Congratulations! However, I'm about guide you on how to transform your simple water kefir into flavorful tonics that will awaken your taste senses.

It is possible to add flavorings into your water-kefir, without having to do the second fermentation. It is not an essential process, but it is it is worth the effort.

For the secondary fermentation, you'll need to use air-tight containers or bottles. It is possible to make use of mason jars as well as the standard lids, however, be sure not to let the Kefir water touch the lid made of metal. I strongly suggest using flip-top bottles made of grolsch.

Attention There is a possibility of an explosion in the process of secondary fermentation. To prevent this danger, you must follow these guidelines:

Make sure that your water kefir is at least one inch beyond the cap on the container.

You should drink your water kefir one time each day for 24 hours.

Step One - Adding Fruit, Fruit Juice, or Flavor Extracts

The first step is to decide on the flavor you wish to add to your water Kefir. There are a lot of options to choose from.

Fruit that is fresh: If you're using fresh fruit, cut, slice , or crush it prior to crushing it. This will allow it to give it more flavor and juice. It is important to remove or replace fresh fruit once every hour. The reason is that some fruit tend to become slimy in the water kefir for many hours. I suggest using only organic fruits. The more fresh, the more delicious!

dried fruit: If using dried fruits, you must be careful. Check that all dried fruit that is utilized in the kefir water is free of sulfites, additives, and preservatives.

The juice of fruit can make nearly any juice you'd like. Concentrated juices of fruit are fine However I would recommend using natural juices made from whole fruits. Lakewood Organic Juices(tm) makes amazing organic fruit juices that are bottled.

Extracts of flavor: A lot of people add flavor extracts to their water Kefir. The most popular is likely the finest vanilla extract. It is possible to create the flavor of cream soda in water Kefir.

Spices: You can include certain spices in your water Kefir. I strongly recommend ginger, however, you can also try tea leaves, cinnamon sticks lemon verbena, or dried lavender. Enjoy yourself!

The quantity of fruit that you include in your water kefir is entirely yours to decide. The more sugar is present of the flavorings you use and the longer time you need to allow all the sugars to ferment and then ferment. We'll discover some fantastic recipes after this chapter, which you can make your ratios based on.

Step Two - Secondary Fermentation

After you have picked out your juices, fruits and extracts, or spices; you're ready to continue through the process.

Secondary Fermentation

Add your juices, fruits, etc. into your water kefir.

Make sure you cap your water kefir to ensure that it is airtight.

Place your water kefir in your normal spot for approximately 24 hours.

Within 24 hours transfer your water kefir into the refrigerator.

Keep your water kefir in the refrigerator for 24 to 72 hours.

You can take your time enjoying the process!

A reminder to drink your water kefir each 24 hours.

30 Delicious and Amazing Recipes That Will Change Everything

Each of the recipes below are based on the ratios of the ingredients that are used in around one quarter cup of water Kefir. Be aware that water kefir can be extremely adaptable; experiment and be creative.

Lemonade Water Kefir

1 tbsp. organic lemon juice

Limeade Water Kefir

1 tbsp. organic lime juice

Blueberry Lemonade Water Kefir

A tiny handful of organic, frozen or fresh blueberries

1 tbsp. organic lemon juice

Berry Citrus Water Kefir

4 or 5 organic fresh or frozen blueberries

3 or 4 organic, fresh or frozen raspberries

3 or 4 organic, fresh or frozen blackberries

2 to 3 organic fresh or frozen strawberry
(smashed or chopped)

1 tbsp. organic lime juice, organic lemon

Cherry Lemon-Lime Water Kefir

Around 8 organic fresh cherries (pitted)

1 tbsp. organic lime juice

1 tbsp. organic lemon juice

Strawberry Lemon-Lime Water Kefir

4 to 5 frozen or fresh organic strawberries,
1 tbsp. organic lime juice or organic lemon

Strawberry Peach Lemonade Water Kefir

4 or 5 organic fresh or frozen strawberries

2 or 3 tablespoons. Fresh organic pureed peach (or juice)

1 tbsp. organic lemon juice

Strawberry Kiwi Lemonade Water Kefir

4 or 5 organic, fresh or frozen strawberries

Half organic Kiwi (chopped)

1 tbsp. organic lemon juice

Tropical Blast Water Kefir

1 tbsp. Organic pineapple juice

1 tbsp. Organic orange juice

1 tbsp. organic lime juice

Cranberry Pomegranate Water Kefir

Organic cranberries in 6 or 7 sizes

1 tsp. organic lime juice

1 tbsp. organic juice of pomegranate

Cranberry Lemonade Water Kefir

10 organic the cranberries

2 tbsp. Organic lemon juice

Strawberry Hibiscus Water Kefir

Fresh or frozen organic strawberries (chopped)

1/2 tbsp. Organic leaves of hibiscus

1 tsp. organic lime juice

Orange-Carrot Water Kefir

1 tbsp. organic carrot juice

1 tbsp. Organic orange juice

Mint-Citrus Orange Water Kefir

1 tbsp. organic lime juice

1 tbsp. Organic orange juice

1 tablespoon fresh Organic mint leaves (chopped)

Minty Mango Water Kefir

2 tbsp. natural mango (or juice)

1 tbsp. Fresh Organic mint leaves (chopped)

Mango Pineapple Colada Water Kefir

2 tbsp. Organic mango (or juice)

2 tbsp. fresh fruit (or juice)

1 tbsp. organic lime juice

Vanilla Cream Soda Water Kefir

2 tsp. organic high-quality vanilla extract

1 tsp. Organic sugars of your preference

Creamy Orange Soda Water Kefir

2 tsp. organic high-quality vanilla extract

2 tbsp. Organic orange juice

Ginger Lemon Water Kefir

1 tbsp. organic lemon juice

1 tbsp. freshly ground organic ginger (or less, based on your personal preferences)

1/2 tbsp. organic lemon zest (optional)

Citrus Pomegranate Water Kefir

1 tbsp. Organic grapefruit juice

1 tbsp. Organic orange juice

1 tbsp. organic juice of pomegranate

2 tsp. organic lemon juice

1/2 tsp. organic orange zest (optional)

1/2 tsp. organic lemon zest (optional)

Peachy Melon Water Kefir

1 tbsp. organic honeydew

1 tbsp. Organic cantaloupe

1 tbsp. organic peach

1 tsp. organic lime juice

1 tsp. organic lemon juice

Peachy Lemonade Water Kefir

2 tbsp. Organic fruit juice (or juice)

1 tbsp. organic lemon juice

Blackberry Lavender Water Kefir

5 organic, fresh or frozen blackberries

2 tsp. fresh lavender (or less, depending on your personal preferences)

Melon Mint Cucumber Water Kefir

2 tbsp. Organic honeydew

2 tbsp. Organic cucumber

1 tbsp. freshly cut organic mint leaves

Blueberry Coconut Water Kefir

1/4 cup coconut water that is organic and made from coconut

10+ organic, fresh or frozen blueberries

Cranberry Apple Water Kefir

1/4 cup of organic Cranberry juice

Organic apple 1/4-cup (chopped or cut)

Grape Water Kefir

1 cup of organic juice from grapes or of organic grapes (chopped)

Creamy Ginger Spice Water Kefir

(for for this dish, make use of ginger in your primary fermentation)

1/2 tbsp. organic high-quality vanilla extract

1 cinnamon stick made from organic

Raspberry Mango Water Kefir

1 cup organic mango (chopped) (or juice)

1/2 cup of organic raspberries

Grape Apple Lemonade Water Kefir

2 tbsp. Organic grape juice

1 cup organic apple (chopped or cut)

1 tbsp. organic lemon juice

These recipes are designed to help you start. You can make these recipes using virtually any fruit juice, spice, or extract you'd like.

Storing Water Kefir Grains

You're now aware of all there is to learn about the process of making and fermenting water kefir from background to the creation of delicious, delicious tonics. But what happens if you decide to break from making water Kefir?

In the case of storing grains of water kefir there are two ways I suggest: dehydrating or storing them in sugar water.

Storing in Sugar-Water

(approx. three weeks, or less)

Make sure to heat one quarter cup of water that is high-quality and safe.

Dissolve 1 cup of sugar in the water.

The sugar-water should be chilled until it is at or near the temperature of room.

Add sugar-water kefir water grains to.

Place a lid that is secure (air-tight) onto the container, then place it in the fridge.

If you decide to brew your water kefir once more (within three weeks) then follow this simple procedure: Remove the water kefir grains out of the sugar-water, wash your kefir grains in water and then culture the sugar-water the same way.

Note: It could need a few brews in order for those water kefir grains alive and active.

Dehydrating Water Kefir Grains

(approx. six months, or less)

Rinse your kefir water grains using high-quality water.

Set the grains on non-bleached paper.

The grains should be placed in a secure place.

The grains can be dried at the room temperature for about 3-5 days.

Place the dry kefir grains in a clear plastic, airtight bag.

Seal the bag and place it in the refrigerator.

Take note that you can make use of a dehydrator to dry your grains. Do not let grains get heated past 85degF. This is slightly more dangerous, but it is possible to do. Make sure you are cautious when doing this.

If you choose to make water kefir once more (within six months) adhere to the rehydration procedure that we discussed within the section "Brewing Your First Batch of Water Kefir".

Note: It could require a couple of brews for your water kefir grain alive and active.

There are some who have successfully frozen their water Kefir grains. I don't suggest this since I've never tried this technique.

Frequently Asked Questions About Water Kefir

Q How much water kefir do I need to drink every day?

A: Before beginning an exercise routine or eating something new initially, you should do it in small quantities. In the end, you can drink as much as want or think you need. Personally, I have around 4 ounces at least twice a every day. Most often, I drink it in between or following meals.

There are some who drink as much as 4 cups daily! The key is balance and moderation. When you first begin to consume water kefir, it could be difficult because of its acidic nature alcohol content, its high probiotics, or just the carbonation. Be patient and let your body adjust to it.

Q What is the process by which water kefir grains grow the sugar-water?

A: The water kefir grains are a symbiotic group of yeast and bacteria that are fed by the natural sugars that are present in your water mix as well as the fruits you consume. The yeast and bacteria within the water kefir grains work together, transforming the nutrients that are not accessible into nutrients that can be accessed by one another. The result is a beverage which has all of its sugars transformed into simpler sugarslike the acetic and lactic acids, CO_2 and alcohol.

The beverage is also rewarded with probiotics in the millions. It also creates bio-available and digestible nutrients by consuming the fruits, sugars and juices, including numerous B vitamins as well as vitamin C.

Q: I have a candida-related issue. Is drinking water kefir a safe thing to drink?

The answer is Candida is an atypical yeast-like fungus. Many sufferers are suffering from candida-related ailments. There have been numerous cases of people with candida-related issues claiming that drinking the benefits of drinking water kefir! Kefir water and the water kefir grains don't contain candida albicans, and there is no reason to cause adverse reactions for those suffering from candida-related ailments. Many of the contributors in the holistic movement have stated that yeast from water kefir can possibly reduce candida yeast. It is essential to learn about your body's signals and to listen to the signals and signs it provides you with.

Q Do water kefirs contain alcohol?

A: Yes. Research has concluded that water kefir has between .03 percent or 2% alcohol. It is approximately .08 per cent on average during the 48-hour fermentation. Kefir made from water that has been kept in storage or allowed to ripen for a few days can have more than that, about 3 percent. Amount of alcohol that kefir produces is limited by the acetic bacteria.

Q How do my water kefir grains appear?

A: The grains of water kefir are semi-transparent. They are available in a broad variety of dimensions and shapes. They could change according to various seasons. They can range from small and uniform in appearance to becoming big and bulky. The colour of your water kefir grain may also differ. They'll always be semi-transparent However, the color will change based on the ingredients and sugars you employ.

Q I have a question: My water kefir grain are floating. Is this normal?

A: Sure! My floats are always on. The majority of water kefir grains hold onto a portion from the CO2 gas that yeast release during the process of fermentation. Some grains are just lower density than sugar water that causes them to sink. Most of the water kefir grain will sit at the bottom of the vessel during the process of fermentation.

Question: Am I need to be careful when handling my water kefir grain?

A No, it's not actually. The water kefir grains are robust. They'll break down as time passes when exposed them to more stress, however they will always recover if living conditions are perfect. The grains of water kefir can withstand situations like mixing with stirring or beaten with the sledgehammer, freezing and drying... but not cooking or using a large quantity of heat. But, be sure to take treatment of the water kefir grain and they'll continue to provide you with the best care.

Q I have a question: My water kefir grain aren't growing, is there something wrong?

A Note: Just because the grains of water-kefir haven't been increasing in number doesn't mean they're unhealthy or have been spoiled. They can still produce sugar-water in a healthy way. To promote the growth and growth that you have in your water-kefir grain Try increasing your water's mineral count by increasing the amount of minerals utilized and providing them with the best conditions to thrive.

A: Should I need to use organic products when making water Kefir?

A: Well, no. Organic products generally contain fewer preservatives, additives and are sprayed with toxins. For instance lemons don't have been organic to qualify as such. You can simply avoid using the rind since that's where the toxic sprays and waxes can be discovered. The water kefir grains react in a way that is based on the quality of the sugar inside the ingredient, and not on whether they are organic or not. All that said I highly recommend using organic, fresh and non-GMO items.

Q What is the appropriate way to use fresh vegetables? I use fresh veggies as my main fermentation?

A: Sure! The water kefir grains are fond of root vegetables like ginger or carrots because of the higher mineral and sugar content. I highly suggest playing with ginger and carrots in your dishes. Don't use other foods such as garlic or onions due to their antibacterial qualities.

Q: How do I make my water kefir become more fizzy?

A: Easy! Once you have completed your second fermentation (24hrs) you can place your water kefir in an airtight container and put it in the refrigerator for up to 2-4 days. You should leave one inch of space between the cap, and then burp it every hour for 24 hours. This will not affect the volume of fizz in the final product.

Q: I did not strain my water Kefir! Do my water kefir grainy flakes in good condition?

A: They'll be very fine. Kefir grains made from water are extremely tolerant. Simply strain them and feed them the way you would normally. They'll likely be content for the next meal and might make sugar-water at a much faster rate than you would normally. Be sure to keep your eye on them and do not be afraid to give it a try in your first 24-hour period. If you haven't strained the kefir and it's gone over by a week, your Kefir grains might need to be rebalanced. This means you'll require brewing one or two batches before they can start to thrive once more.

Q How long do I need to drink my water kefir that I have made?

A Ideally, you would like to drink your water kefir within 2 weeks. After two weeks, it's completely safe to consume your chilled water Kefir. It might become slightly alcohol-based and may have a distinct taste however it's suitable to drink.

Q: I've forgotten the water kefir I made, and the kefir is now really old. What do I do now?

The water kefir is able to remain for a very long period of time. It could develop a unpleasant smell, similar to pickles or wine. Remove them from their existing sugar-water, wash them with high-quality drinking water and then start a fresh batch of sugar-water that is fresh. They'll probably need some time to cultivating sugar-water to be active once again. If they're still not culturing sugar-water or you think that something is not right, then restart the process. It is likely that a friend is running a great batch or you have a backup of water Kefir grains.

Q What happens if water kefir is cross-contaminated?

A: It's an option. To avoid this, make sure that all of your water kefir products are only used to make water kefir. If this isn't possible you should make sure they're thoroughly cleaned and disinfected prior to using them in conjunction with your water kefir. If you think that cross-contamination, you can use this method to strain your water kefir grains, wash them in high-quality water, rub them between your fingers to eliminate any external contamination that has accumulated and then place them into a jar with only the finest water. Then let them sit inside the water for 24 to 48 hours. Then do a second strain and rinse, and then begin a new batch, and also culture some sugar-water. The process could require repeating at least a couple of times to ensure that cross-contamination is removed.

A: It is ok to eat grain of water kefir?

A: Absolutely! They're almost tasteless however they are healthy and beneficial for the body. They're full of probiotics. In terms of consumption of water Kefir grains, there are two options of drying them out, serving them in salads or drying them out before making them into a powder or adding them to your smoothies of choice. I suggest adding them to your smoothies. There are a few studies that show the water kefir grains contain anti-inflammatory, anti-tumor or even blood pressure equalizing qualities! You can try drinking one-quarter cup per day for brief durations. It's obviously to treat ailments. It's essential to maintain a moderate approach when it comes to practices like this Always listen to your body!

Is it possible for my pet be fed water kefir grains?

A: Sure! Probiotics are beneficial to our pets in the same way that they do for us. Your pet might or not like the water Kefir grains. Be sure to watch the grains and note any reactions they may experience.

Q The water-kefir I was drinking spit out grain in the kitchen counter the floor. Do they have to be cleaned up?

A: This has happened frequently in my own life. Be sure to wash thoroughly with water of high-quality and rub it gently using one of your (clean) fingertips. If you're not happy with the idea of this does not suit you, simply throw the grains of water kefir into the drain.

Q: I suspect that I could be experiencing an adverse reaction from drinking my water kefir. ...?

Q: In the event that you think you're experiencing an allergic or unintentional reaction to drinking water kefir, you should stop immediately and seek out an experienced medical expert. It is very uncommon for allergic or adverse reactions to happen, however it's still possible.

Q Is drinking water kefir made anyone sick?

A One thing I've noticed is that in all my extensive study of water kefir and its consumption, I've not once seen a case of someone getting sick after drinking water Kefir. Numerous studies have proven that the symbiotic colonies of yeasts and bacteria (SCOBY) comprised of water kefir grains battle against invaders like the harmful yeasts, mold, and harmful bacteria.

What is Milk Kefir?

Kefir is fermented in a creamy, cultured milk drink that has remarkable health benefits. Its tart, sour and refreshing flavor is like the consistency and taste of yogurt, however it has more beneficial yeast and probiotic bacteria than yogurt. To fully comprehend how milk gets transformed into kefir it is essential to comprehend the process of fermentation. To allow a process of fermentation to begin, bacteria yeast are added to the substance. For dairy kefir yeasts and yeasts are incorporated into gelatinous grains with different shapes ranging from one rice grain up to formations that are up to an inch in size. When kefir grains get placed in milk, the bacteria begin taking in sugars (lactose in the case of milk) within the milk, that in turn causes the yeast grow and reproduce. It is a microscopic fungus that reproduces through budding and can convert the sugar to carbon dioxide as well as alcohol (its quantity of 1 percent is often ignored). The process of fermentation extends the longevity of the product, increasing the flavor and enhancing the digestibility.

If the body's the proper lactase activity does not occur, lactose flows to the colon unabsorbed and because of the fermentative action of the bacterium, individuals might experience cramps, diarrhea and stomach discomfort. This is known in the medical term "Lactose intolerance" or "lactase deficiency." For those who are lactose-intolerant, kefir's wealth of beneficial yeast and bacteria provides lactase which is an enzyme that eliminates the majority of lactose that is left over after the cultivation process. Within the small intestine the lactase enzyme is released to the digestive tract through the exit from the villi of the intestinal that are located inside the intestine's wall. The enzyme then cleaves lactose from the glycosidic linkage by adding a water-soluble molecule and cutting lactose into two primary components, galactose and glucose, both of which are easily taken up by cells for metabolism and production of energy. Also, kefir grains convert milk with high lactose product into a lower lactose kefir product that is extremely easy for the body to process since its constituent molecules don't have a complex structure and require less processing for our body.

The same procedure that works to hydrocarbons also applies to proteins. Kefir's complete proteins are digested in part by the activity of the grains in kefir and thus more readily utilized in the body of the individual. Tryptophan is one of the amino acids that is abundant in kefir is well-known for its calming effect on the nervous system.

Alongside the beneficial yeast and bacteria, kefir also contains essential amino acids and minerals that aid in maintaining and healing functions. due to the high amount of magnesium and calcium as well as other essential minerals that are essential for the health of your nervous system. Kefir consumption is known to have a significant calm effect on the nerves. Kefir is a great source of phosphorus. It is the second-most abundant mineral that we have in our bodies. It assists us to make use of fats, carbohydrates as well as proteins for cells' growth, maintenance and energy. Kefir is high of Vitamin B12, B1, and Vitamin K. It is a great supply of biotin, which is an B vitamin that assists in the body's absorbing of other B Vitamins including pantothenic acid and folic acid. The many benefits of having an the proper B vitamin intake span from control of liver, kidneys, and nervous system, to aiding in the treatment of skin conditions increase energy levels and boost longevity.

Kefir's benefits when consumed often in your eating plan is numerous. It is easy to digest, cleanses the intestines, offers beneficial yeast and bacteria as well as vitamins and minerals and full protein. Kefir is an nutrient-rich and balanced food, it helps to maintain the health of your immune system. It can be used to aid sufferers with AIDS as well as the chronic fatigue syndrome (CFS), herpes and cancer. The calming effect it has over the nerve system been beneficial to many people suffering from depression, sleep disorders and Attention deficit hyperactivity disorder. Kefir's use regularly will help alleviate all intestinal problems, encourage digestion, lessen flatulence and promote better digestion. Furthermore its cleansing effects across the entire body assists to create a healthy inner system for optimal longevity and health. Kefir is also able to help reduce unwholesome food cravings, by helping to keep the body well-nourished and balanced. Kefir's rich nutritional content can provide health and healing benefits to those suffering from all types of health condition. This is due to its focus on digestion, which is the walls of the intestines , where around 80percent part of our immunity lives according to numerous studies. The GI tract has a large surface, and can hold two to 3 pounds of bacteria within an adult human body. this is a significant quantity of bacteria that reside in the GI tract. The whole body may experience an enormous difference in the way it functions if the GI system is well-maintained.

It is possible to ask your self, why you don't buy a kefir at an upscale grocery store and not make it yourself? There's no easy answer. There are many factors to take into consideration is to appreciate the amazing distinction between these two products. The significant difference is resulted from the quantity of probiotics that are consumed. In homemade kefir. This amount is a huge difference compared to one you buy from a supermarket. Kefir that is made by the process of live grains contains more than 50 kinds of probiotics, in contrast to commercial kefir where the most they claim is only 12 probiotics. Think about it, the majority Kefir sold in commercial items are limited in how the process of making kefir has to be standardized and controlled. Certain companies have a "mother batch' that contains live grains. They use kefir to be used as the starting point (instead from the grain) in order to create their own kefir. Some blend carefully selected yeast strains and bacteria to replicate the taste of real Kefir. Although both are healthy alternatives, you're not receiving the full range and full power the homemade kefir made with live kefir grains. It is also more expensive for the commercial version, which is not as beneficial in comparison to the homemade. The price difference could amount to $750 per year when a single user drinking two cups of kefir every day is thought to be. In this way, you could make a quick calculation. The only expense for making kefir at home is a entire milk

($3.50 per gallon) which would mean that the annual costs of $160. If someone decides to consume commercial kefir, which is 2 cups daily for a whole year and the cost for a container (4 cups) is $5, the total consumption over a one year could be 182 bottles of purchased kefir, and in dollars equivalent to $910. The odds are favoring homemade kefir, which costs $160 for an ongoing supply of more than 50 probiotics in your body as opposed with $910 to purchase a product that has only a small positive impact.

How to Make Milk Kefir at Home

After having highlighted the advantages of milk kefir, we are eager to go over how to make homemade probiotics that will benefit your health. Kefir production is a process that is cyclical with an average of 20-24 hours, depending on the surrounding temperature. The procedure itself is easy and doesn't need much time, space, or tools. We'll review the process and tools using my examples; yours may be different or differ. We will focus on the suggestions to follow and points to avoid while we work through the tools and procedure.

The Tools You Need

fermenting (storage) storage containers. I recommend using transparent plastic containers or glass jar for greater visibility and understanding of what is happening. It is crucial to be able to see the bottom in the container. As the fermentation process goes in progress, CO_2 gas pockets may be seen on the walls and if you notice them, it signifies that the fermentation process is complete. You might require a container of the same kind or at the very least, of the similar capacity to filter and store the fermented kefir.

The lid or cover on the fermentation vessel should be used to safeguard the kefir grains from dehydration as well as to prevent excessive contact with the air in order to keep yeasts and components out of contact with the culturing medium. There is no need to cover the container with a lid, let carbon dioxide gas out. However, you might want to seal container tightly by storing it in kefir to extend its shelf longevity.

Stirring spoon. I would recommend using a solid spoon to move the grains while straining the kefir. It will help to accelerate the process.

Mesh made of nylon or plastic strainer. I recommend that you keep Kefir grains or fermenting substances from contact with metal object (except stainless steel). Contact with metal could alter the Kefir grains' PH. I recommend nylon or plastic strainers, as they provide a an easier touch on the grain.

After the system is set, let's look at an overview of two primary components, the kefir grains as well as milk. If you follow the normal culturing process following the suggested guidelines the grains will stay in good condition and you do not need to do anything special aside from repeating the fermenting process regularly as well as straining kefir, and then providing your grains by providing fresh, healthy milk. According to the section on history in this book, historically, goat, cow or horse milk was used for making Kefir. This book I'll concentrate on the most widely accessible cow's milk. It's fine to make use of the regular whole milk you buy from your local grocery store. The homogenized and pasteurized milk is perfect for an excellent result. There is no need to look for organic or raw milk products. However, it's recommended to steer clear of dairy products that are fat-free in the process of making kefir unless you really want it. If you use milk that has lower than 3% may cause kefir to become less creamy.

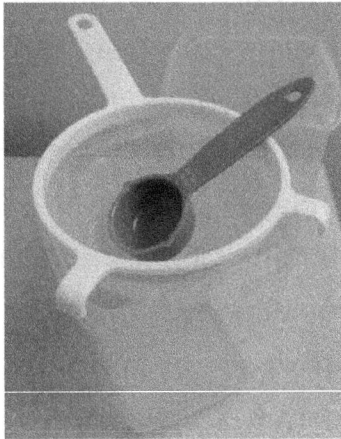

After the grains, milk, and set-up are ready and set, we can move on to the next step.

1. If you calculate that you have the equivalent of one cup of grains of kefir place the milk into the container that is

designated for cultivation process. Incorporate the grains into the milk, or add the grains in the first place; this won't alter the process.

2. Cover the surface of the vessel, then put it in a place in a place where the temperature can be consistently maintained throughout the time needed to finish the fermentation. A good temperature balance should be in the range of 72 to 77F. The container should be left to rest for 20 to 24 hours, while checking periodically. To check if the fermentation is complete, check to see "gas pockets" on the walls of the lower portion in the vessel. If we notice the pockets form and we can tell that Kefir is fermenting and it's moment to strain and break it up from grains. If the time has over, and curds are separated from the whey, creating two layers, simply give the

mixture a vigorous stir prior to straining, and follow the steps as described below.

3. The straining process is straightforward. Place the strainer in an empty container. Pour a small amount of grain and kefir into the strainer. Assist in the process of straining by gently moving the substance through the strainer using the spoon made of plastic. You will notice the slimy consistency of Kefir, also known as the kefiran. It's a sign of good bacteria flourishing. Repetition the fermentation process over small portions until the entire fermented product has been completely removed away from the grains. It is not recommended to clean the grains right now to use kefir grains that are covered with curds to make a new batch. This can help start a new cycle. Then you can run the entire cycle over and over. The fermentation vessel is able to be cleaned

prior to the next time you use it (in this instance, it has to be dried using a tissue paper). If you do not clean your container before using it, this could make fermentation speed up.

Simple guidelines to follow when making kefir by fermenting milk:

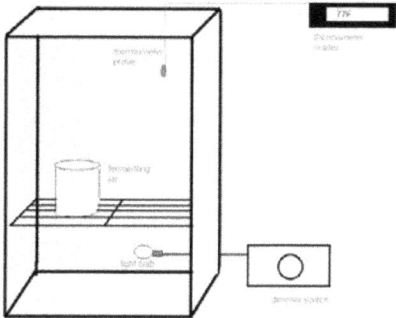

Beware of temperature fluctuations that are out of the suggested norms within the region in which the container to be fermented is located. Keep it out of the oven in the kitchen when not in the kitchen, and keep it out of the windows as a sunny day's temperatures can vary significantly in the evening, and colder temperatures can reduce temperatures in the vessel.

Avoid direct sunlight onto the container due the negative impact that ultraviolet radiation could have on the grains.

Do not let any other metal, besides stainless steel, to touch the fermenting or grainy substance to prevent PH imbalance.

A substance fermented by a strain when first gas pockets are seen to give better results and a more creamy Kefir.

- Don't let kefir grains starve. Do not allow fermented kefir sit with the grains inside it after the curds have been separate from the Whey. In these situations, the grains are starved and don't have lactose in order to feed themselves.

For an effective fermentation, it is essential to keep the temperature within 72F to 77F. What if it's difficult to keep this temperature differential in a location like a mountain house during winter or a the summer heat without air conditioning? In homes located in moderate climates? Temperatures could drop down to 65F for six to twelve hours per day, or higher than 80F. It is likely that you have personal experience that temperatures can increase or decrease significantly when you turn off or shut the temperature of your home's heating or air conditioning during the time that people are off at school or work to reduce energy costs. What can you do to fix the temperature imbalance and offer the grains with an environment that is ideal to ferment? There are solutions to both of these issues.

To maintain the suggested temperature of the the fermenting jar in a cold climate, you could use or construct a wooden box with approximate dimensions W15"xH25"xD10". Install an electrical system with a 25 Watt lamp, dimming switch, and digital thermometer with an external probe. The light bulb should be positioned at the lower part of the box, and power may be controlled by a an dimmer switch located outside the box. The thermometer reader must be placed outside, and its probe is inside the box, around the top.

Take into consideration the safety of your family and security in building this enclosure or using electric installations.

The way to deal with the hot and humid environment where temperatures are always above 85F, and can reach 100F that can harm the health of Kefir grains is to keep the grains in a an isolated area with temperatures in the range of recommended levels, which is slightly lower than 77F. For this it is necessary to use an Styrofoam cooler is a good option. Put ice in containers such as small plastic bottles filled with water or a reused ice-pack container within the cooler. Utilize a thermometer that is digital and remote probes to monitor the temperature. Place the fermenting vessel within the Styrofoam cooler, making sure it isn't touching the containers for ice. Place a thermometer probe into the seal and close it. Allow it to sit for around 20 minutes for the temperature to be stable inside the container and then read the thermometer on the outside. You can alter your temperature with the addition or taking away the containers of ice. Don't use the ice that is in cubes to prevent melted water from touching the fermentation containers. Be aware that it can take a while to see the temperature change inside the box , so be sure to take a look at the thermometer's for a few minutes after. Based on the size of the cooler and outside temperature you'll have to replenish your the ice container at least every few hours during the day. Every circumstance will be different therefore be sure to keep your check on the box until you can figure out how often and in what amount to the circumstances.

Kefir can be kept in the fridge for several weeks without harm to the product. This could be due to nature of harmful microbes are not able to be found in colonies of a healthy bacteria. Certain sources call this the shelf life of a month of Kefir. When storing kefir in a container, ensure that the lid is sealed This will help keep its flavor intact.

How to Take Care of Kefir Grains

If the recommended process and the guidelines above follow when the recommended procedure and guidelines are followed, the kefir grain colony will flourish and remain healthy. But, if the grains were exposed to extreme conditions, such as long storage in a refrigerator, were shipped via mail, or have been left in milk and starved of lactose over a prolonged amount of time they'll need to be revived. To fully reap the benefits for the grain, you'll require an revival process by placing Kefir grains in smaller quantities of milk and changing it more often in shorter intervals to let the grains recuperate. You might want to change the milk every day regardless of whether the fermentation process is completed or not. The straining milk should remain in the refrigerator and not consumed. In the worst cases, this process can last up to three days, however the process described above for a couple of days will usually suffice.

If you're taking the grains out for up to seven days you can put the process of fermentation to a halt by placing the grains in a large amount of milk and then storing it in a refrigerator. The process of fermentation slows down as the temperature decreases. The process can be restarted after you've returned. If you wish to delay the production of kefir for a longer time, rinse them with clear, non-chlorine water, and then keep them in a jar filled with spring water and store them in the refrigerator. This way, the grains can be in storage for up to a month. Once you're ready for making use of them again for fermentation assist the grains to improve their strength by putting the milk in at room temperature until the curds are formed and separation of the whey takes place. Then , strain the milk that was used for the recovery process into the sink and pour in fresh milk to make a delicious Kefir. In order to allow for more storage, kefir grain can be frozen and dried. This treated grain could be kept for up eleven weeks , and then reclaimed in the following week. Remember that regaining grains that have been frozen may require additional effort and takes time. Kefir grains are able to withstand multiple freezing cycles.

Kefir Diets for Losing Weight

Kefir is a healthy and nutritionally dense product. That is the reason it is an ideal base for a variety of diets. The majority of kefir diets are extremely strict and demanding for the body and they are not recommended to consume them for a prolonged duration of duration. However, they can yield significant results when followed strict.

Note: Prior to the consumption of kefir be sure to consult with a doctor.

Seven days kefir diet

First day: five boiled potatoes, and 30 to 44 oz of Kefir.

2nd day: 100 grams of boiled hen and 30 - 44 grams of Kefir.

3rd Day: 100g of cooked meat, and 30-44 OZ l of Kefir.

Fourth day: 100 grams of boiled fish , and 30 - 44 OZ of Kefir.

5th day: fruits and vegetables with the exception of grapes and bananas, plus 30 to 44 oz of Kefir.

6th day: 30-44oz of Kefir, only.

7th day: Mineral water.

It is not recommended to repetitiate this diet more frequently than six times in eight weeks.

Kefir - apple diet

Every day, six times, repeat eating a glass of kefir along with an apple.

This diet is recommended for three to five days.

Kefir mono-diet

Mono diet refers to the fact that there is just one item within the diet, and that product is Kefir in and of itself. It is possible to drink up to 60 ounces of Kefir every day. The most comfortable way to consume it is splitting your diet over six meals daily.

The diet can last from up to three days.

Kefir - avocado diet

The popularity of this diet is because of the combination of two nutritionally rich foods. Avocado contains microelements and nutrients that aid in maintaining well-being while following the diet. The diet comprises three meals daily when you mix half of an avocado and a glass of milk Kefir. There are three meals you can eat every day. You are also permitted to drink plain kefir two times a day.

The diet can last from up to 5 days.

To improve and get a positive results from your diet, think about a gradual return to eating habits that keep your meals low in energy and free from baked goods such as sweet items, baked goods, and food items that are made of white flour.

Recipes Made With Milk Kefir

Before we move on to our delicious dishes, we must address a key question. Does cooking kill probiotics? The answer is simple. There are some studies that suggest that probiotics that have been treated in milk kefir can be beneficial, but a deeper study on this subject is not within our scope in this publication. The focus will be on recipes that use milk kefir is used in its natural state. But, it can be an important ingredient of baking, for instance in the case of making pizzas or sourdough breads.

Okroshka (Russian Cold Soup)

Ingredients:

A quarter cup of finely cut scallions

1 cup chopped finely Dill

1 small bunch of radishes cut in half, then thinly cut into slices

1 small cucumber, peeled , cut into small pieces

Four large eggs hard-boiled and hardboiled and cut into small dice

2 medium-sized boiled waxy potatoes (red or gold) Cut into small pieces

3 cups plain milk kefir

2 cups of water

Salt and pepper as desired

Directions:

Mix chopped scallions, the dill, radishes, cucumber eggs, potatoes and scallions in a large bowl. Separately,, mix the kefir and water to your the desired consistency is achieved, keeping in mind that the final product is more of a soup than salad. Add milk kefir to the bowl until you reach the desired consistency. Pour the mixture of kefir and water over vegetables, and then season with pepper and salt.

Kefir Spread

Ingredients:

3 cups of milk 3 cups of kefir

Garlic or garden vegetables of your preference. Salmon filled could work well.

Directions:

Make silk or cotton cloth (cheese close isn't tight enough). The Milk Kefir into the cone form and allow it to run for 4 to 6 hours, depending on the thickness you want. Mix or crush ingredients like garlic, vegetables, as well as salmon fillet. Mix both ingredients. It is possible to split the drained cream into different parts and add flavors to the different parts.

Kefir Breakfast

Ingredients:

1 Cup of Milk Kefir

1/4 cup of old-fashioned cereals

1/4 cup mixed dates and raisins

2 tablespoons of honey

Directions:

Mix and combine all ingredients in the bowl. You may add any other kinds of dried fruit or change the quantity of honey.

Strawberry Vanilla Kefir

Ingredients:

1 quart of milk from kefir

1/4 cup strawberries, freshly picked or frozen, sliced and frozen is ideal.

1/2 tsp vanilla extract

Honey for taste

Directions:

Add vanilla, strawberries and sweetener, then stir to mix. Blend with the blender.

Cocoa Spice Kefir

Ingredients:

3 cloves

1 stick of cinnamon

A little bit of the nutmeg

1/4 cup cacao powder

1-quart 1 quart of kefir

sweetener to suit your taste (stevia honey, stevia)

Directions:

Mix cocoa powder in the kefir. Add spices. Add the mixture to the mason jar, and let it sit for another 8 to 12 hours. Remove the cinnamon stick as well as the cloves, and blend the kefir to blend it into a smooth. Add sweetener according to your preference.

Rise & Shine Breakfast Smoothie

Ingredients:

2 1/2 cups kefir buttermilk or yogurt

One whole mango either fresh or frozen

2 handfuls of fresh strawberries or frozen

A couple of frozen bananas

1-3 Tbsp. raw honey

A spoonful of coconut oil

1 Tbsp. freshly crushed flaxseed (optional)

Raw egg yolks (optional)

Coconut Flakes of Coconut

Directions:

Pour your preferred milk cultured in the mixer. Add strawberries, mango bananas, mangoes, and honey(add flaxseed or egg yolks if you wish). Mix until it's smooth. While it's making a smooth blend... you can add the coconut oil. allow it to run for one additional minute. Pour the mix into a tall large glass. Top with coconut pieces.